# Aids to Endocrinology

C000133986

# Aids to Endocrinology

## John C. Stevenson
MB BS, MRCP
Endocrine Unit, Royal Postgraduate Medical School, Hammersmith
Hospital, London, UK

## Pritpal Chahal
BSc, MB BS, MRCP
Department of Medicine, Royal Postgraduate Medical School,
Hammersmith Hospital, London, UK

CHURCHILL LIVINGSTONE
EDINBURGH LONDON MELBOURNE AND NEW YORK 1985

CHURCHILL LIVINGSTONE
Medical Division of Longman Group Limited

Distributed in the United States of America by
Churchill Livingstone Inc., 1560 Broadway, New
York, N.Y. 10036, and by associated companies,
branches and representatives throughout the
world.

© Longman Group Limited 1985

All rights reserved. No part of this publication
may be reproduced, stored in a retrieval system,
or transmitted in any form or by any means,
electronic, mechanical, photocopying, recording
or otherwise, without the prior permission of the
publishers (Churchill Livingstone, Robert
Stevenson House, 1–3 Baxter's Place, Leith Walk,
Edinburgh EH1 3AF).

First published 1985

ISBN 0 443 02968 7

British Library Cataloguing in Publication Data
Stevenson, John C.
 Aids to endocrinology.
 1. Clinical endocrinology
 I. Title   II. Chahal, Prit
 616.4   RC648

Library of Congress Cataloging in Publication Data
Stevenson, John C. (John Curtis)
 Aids to endocrinology.
 1. Endocrine glands — Diseases.   I. Chahal, Prit.
II. Title   [DNLM: 1. Endocrine Diseases.   WK 100 S847a]
RC649.S87   1985   616.4   85-6659

Produced by Longman Singapore Publishers (Pte) Ltd.,
Printed in Singapore

# Preface

In this short book we have presented a framework for the understanding of the specialty which we hope will be of use both to medical students and those taking higher qualifications. An understanding of the physiology of endocrine systems is as essential to the endocrinologist as is anatomy to the surgeon, and we have tried to concentrate on this aspect as an introduction to each disorder. Clinical diagnosis and management can only come from experience, and thus we have given solely guidelines in this respect.

We are most grateful for advice and criticism from many colleagues, but in particular Professor Roger Craig and Doctors Roland Jung, A.C. Burden, Tom Adrian and Lawrence Sandler.

We thank Jane Fallows for the illustrations, and Lori Garten and Anne Marie Mulgrew for their help in the preparation of this manuscript.

London, 1985                                                          J.C.S.
                                                                     P.C.

# Contents

# 1. Molecular endocrinology

## HORMONES: SYNTHESIS, ACTIONS AND FUNCTIONS

|  | *Polypeptide* | *Steroidal/thyroid* |
|---|---|---|
| Synthesis | Stored as inactive polypeptide pro-hormone from which active hormone derived | Usually not stored, synthesized de-novo via several intermediates |
| Plasma half-life | Short (minutes) Not protein bound | Long (hours) Protein binding occurs |
| Metabolism | Rapid degradation to inactive components | Peripheral metabolism may produce more active hormone; slow degradation and excretion |
| Cell membrane permeability | Lipid insoluble — require surface receptors | Lipid soluble and easily traverse cell membranes |
| Receptors | Membrane proteins induce secondary messenger systems e.g. c-AMP/$Ca^{2+}$ etc. ? intracellular receptors | Cytoplasmic and nuclear receptors modulate m-RNA production |
| Effects | (i) Rapid (minutes) e.g. ion or nutrient transport (ii) Gradual (hours) — cell growth, division, protein synthesis, etc. | Gradual (hours to days) |

Catecholamines water are soluble and behave as polypeptide hormones.

## HORMONE SYNTHESIS

### Peptide hormones
Four general groups of peptide hormones:
1. *glycoprotein hormones* (LH, FSH, TSH, HCG)
   - consist of 2 polypeptide subunits — $\alpha$ and $\beta$
   - $\alpha$ subunit common to all — $\beta$ subunits differ
   - carbohydrate residues are added to peptide after synthesis and $\alpha$ and $\beta$ subunit peptides joined
2. *large single-chain hormones* (GH, placental lactogen, PRL, PTH)
   - single polypeptide chain
   - have some amino-acid sequence homology
3. *small multi-chain hormones* (insulin, relaxin)
   - contain 2 non-identical peptide chains
   - chains linked by disulphide bridges
4. *small single-chain hormones* (numerous)
   - large array of sizes
   - often require carboxyl terminal amide for biological activity

Many peptide hormones are synthesized as larger inactive precursors forms.

### Synthesis (Fig. 1.1)
1. *Gene*
   - DNA carries information for synthesis of peptide
   - cleavage sites are indicated by special nucleic acid codes (intron)
   - may be regulators of expression close to site of gene

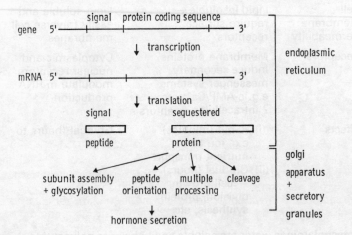

**Fig. 1.1**

- may have more than one gene encoding for peptide (e.g. GH)
- may have one gene encoding for more than one peptide (e.g. pro-opiomelanocortin)
- DNA variations shown by Southern blotting hybridization techniques

2. *Messenger RNA*
   - mRNA is a copy of DNA nucleic acid sequence (transcription)
   - non-coding sequences excluded to form mature mRNA
   - may be post-transcriptional modifications yielding different mature mRNAs (e.g. calcitonin/CGRP)
   - RNA variations shown by Northern blotting hydridization techniques

3. *Precursor polypeptide*
   - ribosomes interpret data carried by mRNA and synthesize peptide with correct order of aminoacids (translation)
   - precursor polypeptide may contain one or more peptide hormones
   - precursor cleaved at predetermined sites as it is being extruded through the endoplasmic reticulum
   - liberated peptides transferred to Golgi apparatus where further cleavage may occur
   - may be post-translational modifications such as glycosylation, phosphorylation, methylation and acetylation to activate hormone
   - may be alternative post-translational cleavage of precursor polypeptides at different sites (e.g. pro-opiomelanocortin)
   - normal/abnormal precursor polypeptides and cleavage fragments shown by specific immunoassay/immunolocalization

4. *Peptide storage*
   - peptide hormones stored in secretory granules until released
   - further cleavage may occur here or peripherally after secretion (e.g. PTH)
   - normal/abnormal circulating peptides shown by specific assay

**Steroid hormones**
- all steroid hormones are based on cholesterol which is metabolized enzymatically
- specific metabolic pathways exist for the production of each steroid hormone
- metabolic pathway of a steroid hormone may be confined to a single endocrine gland e.g. corticosteroids or may require steps in different tissues e.g. vitamin D

## HORMONE RELEASE

neuronal         – in response to neuronal transmission e.g.
                   posterior pituitary hormones,
                   catecholamines
                 – in response to 'higher centres' e.g.
                   hypothalamic releasing factors
biochemical      – in response to changes in circulating levels
                   of certain chemicals e.g. insulin response to
                   glucose
hormonal         – in response to releasing and inhibiting
                   hormones e.g. GH response to GRF and
                   somatostatin
tissue damage    – leakage from damaged endocrine tissue e.g.
                   thyroid hormones in thyroiditis
hormone release  – may be pulsatile e.g. GnRH
                 – may be cyclical e.g. cortisol
                 – may be continuous e.g. thyroxine


## HORMONE ACTIONS

### Receptors
Mechanism of hormone-receptors interaction poorly understood
Hormone will exert effect where target receptors exist
Hormones may share receptors though affinity may be less or
enhanced
Receptors can mediate stimulatory and inhibitory effects

*Cell surface receptors*
On binding to hormone, receptors on cell surface aggregate (?
mediated by contractile proteins — actin, troponin); aggregation
may mediate rapid effects of polypeptide hormones on ion,
nutrient transport
   At sites of aggregation, pinocytosis occurs, which may:
1. aid in regulating membrane receptor population by lysosomal
   degradation
2. allow access of peptide hormone to intracellular organelles or
   nucleus of target cells mediating effects on growth, cell
   division, protein synthesis etc.

### The concept of membrane regulatory proteins (Fig. 1.2)
– Surface receptors are linked to adenyl cyclase by membrane
  regulatory proteins called N or G proteins because they can
  bind Nucleotide, or more precisley GTP. These proteins may be
  closely associated with the receptor.
– On binding of hormone to its receptor, conformational changes
  in the N-protein allow GTP to combine with it. A receptor-N-

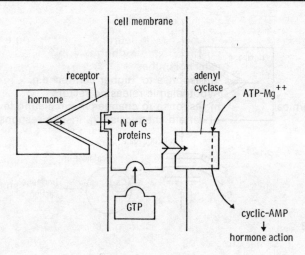

cell membrane

receptor

hormone

N or G proteins

GTP

adenyl cyclase

ATP-Mg$^{++}$

cyclic-AMP
↓
hormone action

**Fig. 1.2**

protein-GTP complex is formed, which can influence adenyl cyclase activity and hence cyclic-AMP production. Cyclic AMP then acts as second messenger. The role of GTP is crucial, as many hormones require its presence for their action.
- Depending on the nature of the receptor, N proteins can be stimulatory or inhibitory on adenyl cyclase activity.
- Activation of some surface receptors opens membrane-bound calcium channels permitting calcium to enter cytosol and act as second messenger.

**Secondary intracellular events**
amplify extracellular signals
*cyclic AMP*
- rising levels activate intracellular protein kinases to phosphorylate cell proteins
- falling levels lead to dephosphorylation of cell proteins
*calcium ions* (Fig. 1.3)
- alter conformation of intracellular calmodulin
- calcium-calmodulin complex activates target proteins

*Abnormalities of N protein function*
Some cases of receptor dysfunction may be due to N protein dysfunction. There is some evidence that pseudohypoparathyroidism, in which there is peripheral unresponsiveness to PTH, and occasionally other hormones, represent N-protein deficiency.

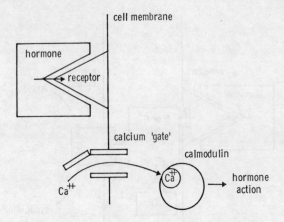

**Fig. 1.3**

*Intracellular receptors*
- lipid soluble steroidal hormones bind to receptor protein in cytoplasm
- hormone receptor complex translocated to nucleus
- hormone-receptor complex interacts with nuclear membrane receptor or intranuclear chromatin receptor to eventually modulate mRNA synthesis
- mRNA may then direct protein synthesis related to metabolic effect of hormone

*Receptor regulation*
- complex hormone and receptor interactions play important role in receptor regulation
- high and prolonged exposure of target cells to hormone can result in biological desensitization via a reduction in receptor numbers — down regulation

*Mechanism of down-regulation not understood:*
- ? increased aggregation and pinocytosis of surface receptor-hormone complex
- ? intracellular messenger dysfunction
- ? decreased receptor synthesis or binding affinity
- ? pattern of hormone release — physiological release of hormone may be pulsatile and allow recovery of receptors to avoid down regulation

*Hormones that induce 'down-regulation'*
TRH/GnRH
GH
Gonadotrophins

Insulin
Glucagon
Calcitonin
Catecholamines
T3
Synthetic hormone agonists
? Steroids
Some hormones increase their receptors i.e. up-regulation —
mechanisms not known, e.g.:
Prolactin
Angiotensin
Oestrogens — also stimulate progesterone receptors
Synthetic hormone antagonists

**Feedback mechanisms**
Target cell hormones may inhibit or stimulate secretion of
hypothalamic or pituitary trophic hormones. Inhibitory influences
may be tonic, involving critical interaction of target cell hormone
with trophic hormone synthesis or release; inhibitory proteins
may be involved in some cases.
   Peripheral polypeptide hormones secretion can be related to
ionic (e.g. PTH and $Ca^{+2}$) or nutrient (insulin and glucose) fluxes
— again feedback control is not understood.

*Endocrine diseases associated with receptor absence or
dysfunction*
In most such diseases trophic hormone is elevated.

| *Receptor deficiency* | *Disease* |
|---|---|
| PTH | Pseudohypoparathyroidism |
| Insulin | Diabetes — Type II |
| GH | Laron dwarfism |
| Vasopressin | Nephrogenic diabetes insipidus |
| Testosterone | Testicular feminization |
| T3 | Hypothyroidism |
| LDL-lipoprotein | Familial hypercholesterolaemia |
| 1,25 dihydroxyvitamin D | Vitamin D-dependent rickets type II |

| *Receptor auto-antibody* | |
|---|---|
| TSH | Autoimmune thyroid disease |
| Insulin | Acanthosis nigricans with insulin resistant diabetes |

**HORMONE FUNCTIONS**

1. *Neurocrine* e.g. substance P
   - hormone released by neurone
   - acts as a neurotramsmitter
   - influences cells in close contact

2. *Paracrine* e.g. GnRH
   - hormone released by non-neural secretory cell
   - influences cells in close vicinity
   - may not enter systemic circulation
3. *Endocrine* e.g. insulin
   - hormone released directly into circulation by specific
     secretory cells
   - secretory cells may form distinct gland
   - influences cells in distant 'target' organs

Some hormones may have some or all of above functions e.g.
somatostatin is a neurotransmitter, a local hypothalamic
inhibiting factor and a circulating hormone.

*Tissue growth factors*
Evidence mostly from animal studies indicates that tissue
development, mitosis and growth is mediated by local and/or
circulating growth factors.
- growth factors are large peptides which act via surface
  receptors on target cells
- may be structurally related to hormones
- some classical hormones can stimulate synthesis and secretion
  of growth factors

*Epidemal growth factor (EGF)*
- located along GI tract, thyroid and kidneys
- identical to urogastrone in humans which inhibits intrinsic
  factor and gastric acid secretion
- stimulated by thyroid and androgen hormones
- ? fetal development
     epidermal cell differentiation, and growth
     stimulates surfactant in lung
- promotes malignant tumour growth

*Nerve growth factor (NGF)*
- source may be cells innervated by sensory and sympathetic
  nerves in which it is present
- stimulated by thyroid hormones
- essential for differentiation, growth and sustenance of sensory
  and sympathetic nerve activity
- ? deficient NGF production may explain familial dysautonomia
- ? excess NGF may stimulate neuroectodermal tumours

*Fibroblast pneuomocyte factor (FPF)*
- occurs in fetal lung fibroblast
- stimulated by glucocorticoids
- important for surfactant synthesis and secretion from type II
  pneumonocyte

*Platelet derived growth factor*
- occurs in platelet α-granules
- may result in vascular smooth muscle and connective tissue proliferation at site of sub-endothelial exposure due to vascular damage e.g. enhance wound repair

## MOLECULAR BIOLOGY TECHNIQUES

*Southern blot hybridization*
- used to investigate DNA
1. DNA digested with appropriate restriction enzymes — yields fragments
2. restriction fragments separated by gel electrophoresis
3. fragments transferred to suitable filter by capillary blotting
4. labelled known DNA sequence (probe) identifies same sequence on filter (hybridization)

*Northern blot hybridization*
- used to investigate RNA to a similar manner to Southern blot hybridazation.

*Nucleotide sequence analysis*

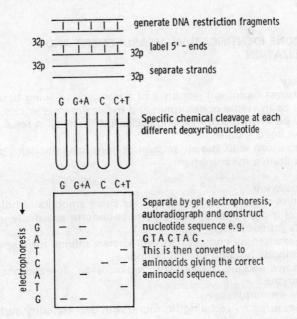

Fig. 1.4

## Cloning

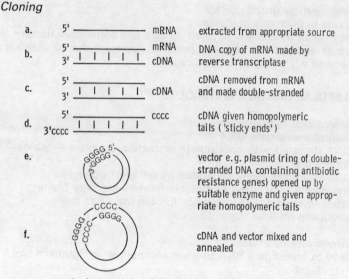

a.    5' ———————— mRNA    extracted from appropriate source

b.    5' ———————— mRNA    DNA copy of mRNA made by
      3' | | | | | cDNA    reverse transcriptase

c.    5' ———————— cDNA removed from mRNA
      3' | | | | | cDNA    and made double-stranded

d.    5' ———————— cccc    cDNA given homopolymeric
      3'cccc | | | | |     tails ('sticky ends')

e.                         vector e.g. plasmid (ring of double-
                           stranded DNA containing antibiotic
                           resistance genes) opened up by
                           suitable enzyme and given approp-
                           riate homopolymeric tails

f.                         cDNA and vector mixed and
                           annealed

g.    vector inserted into suitable host e.g. E.coli and colonies then
      grown, thus reproducing the required DNA.

**Fig. 1.5**

# HORMONE IDENTIFICATION, MEASUREMENT AND LOCALIZATION

## Bioassay
- measures biological response of a hormone in living tissue
- may be in vivo e.g. calcitonin and hypocalcaemia in rats
- may be in vitro e.g. PTH and cyclic AMP activity in renal convoluted tubules
- comparison with known amount of hormone (standard) gives quantitative measurement

## Immunoassay
- permits measurement of extremely small amounts of hormone
- use of monoclonal antibody permits uniform specificity
- 1-site immunoassay
  - measured by competition with known antigen for a specific
  - antibody binding site on hormone
  - known antigen labelled with radioisotope, fluorescence or enzyme
- 2-site immunoassay
  - measured by isolating hormone with one antibody and detecting it with a second antibody labelled with radioisotope, fluorescence or enzyme

*Competitive binding assay*
- measures by competition with known hormone for specific binding sites on carrier protein or receptor
- known antigen usually labelled with radioisotope
- used for steroid hormone measurement

*Mass spectrometry*
- measures mass of molecules and their fragments on the basis of different mass/charge values
- used for structural elucidation of peptides, steroids etc.

*Hormone separation*
- used for isolation, purification, characterization
1. *peptides*
    - gel filtration — separation by size
    - reverse phase HPLC — separation by hydrophobicity
    - ion exchange chromatography — separation by charge
    - immuno-affinity chromatography — separation by antigen specificity
2. *steroids*
    - normal/reverse phase HPLC — separation by hydrophobicity
    - gas chromatography — separation by polarity
    - ion exchange chromatography — separation by charge

*Hormone localization*
- tissue extraction, separation and assay of hormone
- binding to specific immunofluorescent or enzyme-linked antiserum — histological identification
- binding to specific antiserum with attached gold particles — electrom-microscopical identification
- hybridization of specific labelled cDNA probes to mRNA in situ

# 2. Hypothalamic-pituitary disorders

## HYPOTHALAMUS

### Physiology

'Higher' centres

Various neurotransmitters:
- neuropeptides
- adrenergic
- dopaminergic
- cholinergic
- serotoninergic

'Target' hormone feedback ⟶ HYPOTHALAMUS

'Endocrine' functions:
mainly ventromedial

Other functions:
mainly antero-posterior

Sleep/arousal
thermoregulation
thirst
eating
'Autonomic' activity
memory

Direct secretion of

- oxytocin
- vasopressin
- neurophysin

Releasing hormones or factors

- stimulatory
- inhibitors

Axonal transport
of neurosecretory granules

Portal capillary system

POST PITUITARY

ANT PITUITARY HORMONE
SECRETION

- There is a variable degree of anatomical overlap of hypothalamic functions
- Bilateral lesions are required to produce clinically apparent hypothalamic disease
- Ventromedial lesions tend to cause bilateral damage

Endocrine syndromes of hypothalamic dysfunction
- ADH deficiency or increased ADH
- precocious puberty
- variable hypopituitarism (deficiency of releasing hormones)
- ? hypothalamic Cushings disease

Causes of hypothalamic dysfunction:
- Developmental abnormalities
  - agenesis of corpus callosum
  - isolated GnRH deficiency (Kallmans syndrome)
  - familial syndromes e.g. diabetes insipidus
  - chronic hydrocephalus
  - Frohlichs syndrome
- Increased intracranial pressure
- Tumours
    craniopharyngioma
    suprasellar extension of pituitary tumour
    hamartoma
    glioma
    meningioma
    dermoid
    leukaemia/lymphoma
    metastases e.g. breast carcinoma
- Granuloma
    tuberculosis
    sarcoid
    histiocytosis-X
- Infective
    meningitis
    encephalitis
    sphenoid osteomyelitis
- Vascular
    infarction
    aneurysm
    subarachnoid haemorrhage
    A-V malformation
- Degenerative
    demyelinating diseases
    Wernickes encephalopathy
- Trauma
- Surgery
- Cranial irradiation

- Stress
  emotional deprivation
  starvation
- Drugs
  dopamine antagonists
  metoclopramide
  antipsychotics e.g. chlorpromazine, butyrophenol

## PITUITARY TUMOURS

*Causes*
- adenohypophysis
  - chromophobe adenoma
  - acidophil adenoma
  - basophil adenoma
  - mixed adenoma
- craniopharyngioma (see above)
- multiple endocrine neoplasia type I
  - pituitary adenoma
  - hyperparathyroidism
  - pancreatic endocrine tumour
  - adrenocortical tumour
- metastatic tumour (primary malignancy extremely rare)

*Clinical features*
1. *Local effects*
   - compression of optic chiasma — visual field defects (usually temporal quadrantinopia)
   - headache — traction on dura
   - compression of pituitary gland — hypofunction
2. *Systemic effects*
   - due to specific pituitary hormone hypersecretion/hyposecretion

## GENERAL PITUITARY INVESTIGATIONS

### Radiology
1. *plain radiography and tomography*
   - sellar enlargement
   - abnormal sellar shape
   - double contour
   - erosion of floor and clinoids
   - calcification (craniophargyngioma)
2. *CT scanning* (high resolution)
   - demonstrates sella contents
   - demonstrates suprasellar extension
   - non-invasive

**Biochemistry**
1. *measurement of pituitary hormones*
   - direct measurements
   - patterns of release e.g. ACTH
2. *stimulation of pituitary hormones*
   - insulin hyporglycaemia — GH, ACTH
   - TRH — TSH, prolactin
   - GnRH — FSH, LH
   - CRF — ACTH
   - GRF — GH
3. *suppression of pituitary hormones*
   - glucose tolerance test — GH
   - T$_3$ suppression test — TSH
   - dexamethasone suppression test — ACTH
   - oestradiol administration — FSH, LH
4. *measurement of target organ hormone production*
   See relevant chapters

## MANAGEMENT

### Surgery

*Indications*
- large tumours
- significant suprasellar or parasellar expansion
- compression of optic chiasma or foramen of Monro

*Technique*
- trans-sphenoidal (90%)
- transfrontal
- selective microadenomectomy often possible

### Irradiation

*Indications*
- intrasellar adenoma
- little suprasellar or parasellar expansion
- adjunct to surgery

*Technique*
- interstitial irradiation by [90]Yttrium implantation
- conventional radiotherapy

### Medical treatment

*Indications*
- intrasellar adenomas
- prolactinomas
- some cases of acromegaly/Cushing's
- adjunct to surgery/irradiation

*Technique*
- bromocriptine — especially prolactinoma, acromegaly
- sodium valproate — Nelson's syndrome

## PANHYPOPITUITARISM

Partial or total failure of anterior pituitary function

**Causes**
- pituitary adenoma
- Sheehan's syndrome (postpartum necrosis)
- craniopharyngioma
- pituitary infarction
- granuloma
- secondary metastases
- trauma
- surgery/radiotherapy

**Clinical features**
- usually slow onset
- local tumour effects
- effects of hormone deficiency
  - gonadotrophin deficiency
  - TSH deficiency
  - ACTH deficiency
- anaemia (normochromic)
- fine, smooth, pale skin
- deficiency of body hair
- genital atrophy

**Investigations**
General pituitary investigations

**Management**
- restoration of normal hormonal status
- treatment of underlying disorder if possible

## 'EMPTY SELLA'

Variable extension of cerebrospinal fluid-space into pituitary fossa

**Causes**

*Primary*
- commoner in females and in obese
- ? CSF pressure compressing pituitary gland, which forms a rim at bottom of sellae
  - congenital defect of diaphragma sella

- benign intracranial hypertension (occurs in 10% of patients)
- compression of pituitary stalk by 'kinked' internal carotid arteries

*Secondary*
- hypophysectomy
- pituitary irradiation
- spontaneous pituitary tumour infarction

## Clinical features
- incidental finding of abnormal pituitary fossa on skull radiology or computerized tomography (CT)
- headaches (non specific)
- CSF, rhinorrhoea (very rare)
- visual field defects (very rare)
- hypopituitarism occurs with secondary causes; rim of pituitary tissue sufficient to sustain normal endocrine function in primary disease

## Investigations
- symmetrically ballooned pituitary fossa with preservation of clinoids and dorsum sella on radiology suggests primary 'empty sella'
- CT scan with metrizamide scanning will confirm 'empty' sella and also detect a coexisting intrasellar tumour
- pituitary function tests abnormal if secondary causes — usually normal if primary

## Management
- primary disease requires only follow up with checks on endocrine function
- secondary causes may require hormone replacement

## GH (growth hormone)

### Physiology
1. synthesis (acidophil cell) (Fig. 2.1)

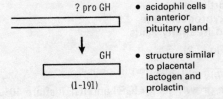

? pro GH    ● acidophil cells in anterior pituitary gland

GH    ● structure similar to placental lactogen and prolactin
(1-191)

**Fig. 2.1**

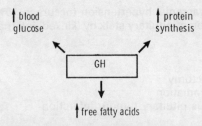

● actions via somatomedin and ? direct

**Fig. 2.2**

2. control — via 2 hypothalamic polypeptides: GRF (growth hormone releasing factor) and somatostatin

Stimulation:

| hypoglycaemia | via |
| glucagon | ventromedial |
| arginine- | nucleus |
| vasopressin | |

| deep sleep | via limbic |
| ? pyrogens | system |

: GH ↑
(via GRF)

stress
exercise
dopamine
oestrogen
serotonin
protein malnutrition
opioids

Suppression:

| hyperglycaemia | via ventromedial |
| β adrenergic stimulation | nucleus |

chlorpromazine via arcuate nucelus

somatomedin
? GH

: Gh ↓
(via somatostatin)

obesity
glucocorticoid
medroxyprogesterone
elevated free fatty acids

3. *actions* (Fig. 2.2)

*Somatomedins* (Fig. 2.3)
– Insulin like growth factor IGF I and IGF II share 40% homology with A and B chains of insulin and all have similar 3-dimensional structure

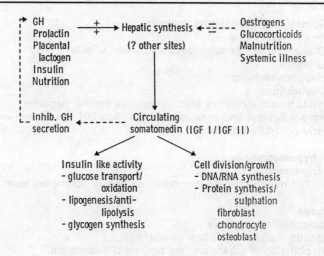

**Fig. 2.3**

- In circulation, somatomedins may bind to specific proteins
- Surface receptors for IGF are similar in structure to insulin receptors
- GH is especially trophic for IGF I which also controls GH secretion by negative feedback inhibition
- Trophic hormone for IGF II not known


*Causes of increased IGF I*
Acromegaly
IgF receptor detect


*Causes of decreased IGF I*
GH deficiency/inactive GH form
Laron dwarfism (GH increased)
- GH receptor defect
- GH synthesis defect
Malnutrition
Hepatic dysfunction
Pygmies (IGF I low with normal IGF II)
Uraemia (but increased IGF II)
Diabetes — but is normal with good control


*Somatomedin inhibitors*
Discrepancy between radioimmunoassay and biological assay studies may be explained by circulating inhibition factors of somatomedin acting at receptor or post-receptor levels. Effects of insulin are also antagonized.

Somatomedin inhibitors occur in:
- Insulin deficiency
- Diabetic states (also antagonize insulin effects)
- Uraemia
- Hypophysectomy
- Malnutrition

Somatomedin inhibitors also antagonize central negative feedback control and may explain the high GH levels seen in poorly controlled diabetes.

**GH hypersecretion**
1. *Gigantism*
   - GH hypersecretion commencing before epiphyses fuse

*Causes*
- acidophil hyperplasia
- pituitary adenoma (often presumed)
- hypothalamic gigantism has normal GH secretion

*Clinical features*
- local tumour effects
- excessive stature for age: exclude constitutional and delayed puberty
- often associated features of acromegaly
2. *Acromegaly*
   - GH hypersecretion after epiphysial fusion

*Causes*
- pituitary adenoma
- rarely acidophil hyperplasia
- ? some cases secondary to hypothalamic dysfunction

*Clinical features*
- onset usually in 4th and 5th decades, M = F
- overgrowth of skeleton
  - skull: frontal sinuses and supraorbital ridges, prognathism
  - vertebrae — kyphosis
  - hands and feet
  - ribs: barrel chest
- overgrowth of skin
  - increased skin thickness
  - exaggerated skin folds
  - excessive sweating
  - seborrhoea
- arthralgia and osteoarthritis
- cardiomegaly: cardiac failure; hypertension
- laryngeal hypertrophy — voice change
- goitre — thyroid function normal

- diabetes mellitus (chemical/clinical)
- carpal tunnel syndrome
- muscle weakness
- gynaecomastia
- galactorrhoea
- hypopituitarism, especially hypogonadism
- local tumour effects

*Investigations*
  General pituitary investigations
- specific - GH levels raised and not suppressed during GTT
  - impaired GTT
  - hypercalcaemia/hypercalciuria
  - skin thickness
    - calipers
    - heel pad X ray
  - hand/foot volumes

*Management*
- surgery
- irradiation
- bromocriptine

## ACTH (adrenocorticotrophic hormone)

### Physiology
1. *Synthesis* (Fig. 2.4)

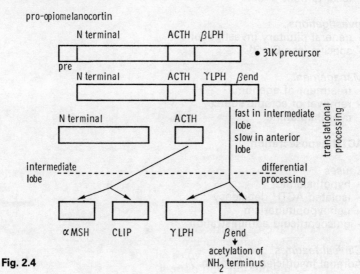

**Fig. 2.4**

2. *Control*
Stimulation:

      glucocorticoid deficiency
      stress

                             via CRF   : ACTH ↑

      hypoglycaemia
      pyrogens

      vasopressin
Suppression:

                                     : ACTH ↓
      glucocorticoid excess

circadian rhythm of ACTH secretion

3. *Actions*
   - increased glucocorticosteroid synthesis and secretion
   - adrenal cortex hyperplasia
   - fat breakdown: free fatty acid release

**ACTH hypersecretion**

*Causes*
- Pituitary adenoma
- ectopic secretion
  - oat cell lung tumour
  - carcinoid

*Clinical features*
- hypercortisolism (see Ch. 7)
- local tumour effects

*Investigations*
- general pituitary investigations
- specific (see Ch. 7)

*Management*
- treatment of adenoma
- removal of ectopic source
- cyproheptadine

**ACTH hyposecretion**

*Causes*
- hypothalamic
- isolated ACTH deficiency
- panhypopituitarism
- glucocorticoid administration

*Clinical features*
Adrenal insufficiency (see Ch. 7)

*Investigations*
- general pituitary investigations
- specific (see Ch. 7)

*Management*
Normalize glucocorticoid status

## NELSON'S SYNDROME

**Definition**
Pituitary ACTH hypersecretion and pigmentation following
bilateral adrenalectomy for pituitary-dependent Cushing's
High incidence (70%) in childhood

*Clinical Features*
- local tumour effects
- skin pigmentation
- previous adrenalectomy
- occasional exophthalmos
- can occur 6 months to decades post-op

*Investigations*
- general pituitary investigations
- specific
    - plasma ACTH often very high
    - often not suppressable

*Management*
Tumour removal
- surgery
- external irradiation
- interstitial irradiation

## ENDOGENOUS OPIATES

- Endogenous opiates are peptides widely dispersed in the body
  with similar pharmacological action to morphine and its
  derivatives.
- Major role may be as modulators, mostly inhibitory, of basal
  neural transmission

**Synthesis and action** (Fig. 2.5)
- Endorphins are derived from β-LPH (β-lipotrophin) segment of
  31K pro-opiomelanocortin molecule.
- Amino acid sequences of enkephalins are present in β-LPH and
  β-endorphins, but actual precursor of enkephalins still not
  characterized.

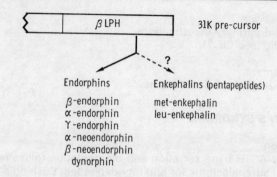

**Fig. 2.5**

- Enkephalins are rapidly inactivated by enkephalinase enzymes; endorphins are also hydrolysed but are more stable.
- Endogenous opiates or their synthetic derivatives poorly traverse the blood-brain barrier, but intra-thecal administration produces profound analgesia.
- Increasing numbers of different receptors are being identified e.g.:
  - $\mu$ (mu) receptor
    - mediates analgesic responses
    - stimulates GH, PRL
    - stimulated by morphine and endogenous opiates especially dynorphin
    - blocked by naloxone
  - $\delta$ (delta) receptor
    - seizure activity, behavioural responses
    - not stimulated by enkephalins
  - $\varepsilon$ (epsilon) receptor — specific for $\beta$-endorphin
  - $\kappa$ (kappa) receptor
    - inhibits vasopressin and oxytocin
    - stimulated by dynorphins, $\beta$-neoendorphin
- Most of the proposed physiological and pathological roles for local endogenous opiates are controversial

**Table 2.1**

| Location of opioid | Opioid type | Possible physiological or pathological role |
| --- | --- | --- |
| *CNS* | | |
| Periaqueductal area | Enkephalins, Endorphins | Modification of pain perception e.g. analgesia by electroacupuncture, placebo, stress, shock etc. |
| Hypothalamus | Enkephalins, Endorphins | Regulation of temperature, satiety, emetic functions of hypothalamus Regulate vasopressin, oxytocin secretion ? inhibitory |
| Limbic, extrapyramidal | Enkephalins, Endorphins | Behavioural response (?disturbed in psychoses) seizures |
| Median eminence | Enkephalins Endorphins | Alter pituitary regulatory hormones to inhibit ACTH, Gonadotrophins, TSH and increase PRL, GH secretions |
| Anterior pituitary | β-endorphin | Released concurrently with ACTH during stress |
| Spinal cord (substantia gelatinosa) | Enkephalin | Modulate perception of pain (? via substance P release) |
| *Other sites* | | |
| Sympathetic ganglia | Enkephalin | Released with catecholamine (? inhibit catecholamine secretion to lower BP) |
| Adrenal medulla | Enkephalin (mostly metenkephalin) | ? role in pathogenesis of endotoxic shock |
| Pancreas | β-endorphin | Stimulates glucagon and insulin secretion |
| Gastrointestinal | Enkephalin | Alters gut motility — increases contractility |

*Causes of increased circulating endogenous opiates*
- endotoxic shock
- chronic renal failure
- ? chlorpropamide alcohol flushing (sherry alone elevates)
- tumours
    - phaeochromocytoma
    - ectopic ACTH
    - other tumours

## TSH (thyroid stimulating hormone)

### Physiology
1. *synthesis* (thyrotroph cell)
    - prohormone not known
    - glycopeptide, similar to FSH, LH
2. *control*
   Stimulation:
     TRH
   Suppression:
     dopamine
     glucocorticoids suppress
     somatostatin
     $T_4$
3. *actions*
    - stimulates
        - iodine transport and trapping
        - thyroid hormone synthesis and secretion
        - thyroid gland hyperplasia

## TSH hypersecretion

*Causes*
- primary hypothyroidism
- pituitary adenoma — very rare

*Clinical features*
- see Chapter 3
- local tumour effects

*Investigations*
- generalized pituitary investigations
- specific (see Ch. 3)

*Management*
- normalize thyroid function
- treat adenoma

**TSH hyposecretion**

*Causes*
- primary hyperthyroidism
- panhypopituitarism

*Clinical features*
- see Chapter 3

*Investigations*
- general pituitary investigations
- specific (see Ch. 3)

*Management*
Normalize thyroid function

**PRL (prolactin)**

**Physiology**

1. *synthesis* (eosinophil cell)
   - structure similar to placental lactogen and GH
   - prohormone not known
2. *control*
   Stimulation:
   - stress
   - suckling
   - oestrogen (including pregnancy)
   - TRH
   - serotonin
   - hypoglycaemia
   - dopaminergic blockers
     - phenothiazines
     - butyrophenones
   - other drugs e.g. morphine, methyldopa, imipramine
   - pituitary stalk section
   Suppression:
   - prolactin inhibitory factor (unknown hypothalamic factor)
   - dopamine + agonists
   - bromocriptine
   - ? VIP, cholecystokinin
3. *actions*
   - breast milk production
   - suppression of menstruation
   - stimulation of 1,25 dihydroxyvitamin D production

## Prolactin hypersecretion

*Causes*
- pituitary adenoma
- pituitary stalk section
- oestrogen
- hyopthyroidism
- dopaminergic receptor blockers e.g. phenothiazines, metoclopramide, methyldopa
- renal failure
- physiological
    - pregnancy
    - breast feeding
    - stress

*Clinical features*
- amenorrhoea
- galactorrhoea   (see Ch. 8)
- osteopenia
- local tumour effects

*Investigations*
- general pituitary investigations
- specific — raised PRL levels

*Management*
- treat adenoma
- bromocriptine

## Prolactin hyposecretion
- panhypopituitarism

## FSH (Follicle-stimulating hormone)

**Physiology**
1. *synthesis* (gonadotroph cell)
    - prohormone unknown
    - glycopeptide, similar to TSH, LH
2. *control*
    Stimulation:
    - GnRH
    - clomiphene
    Suppression:
    - oestrogen
    - progestin
    - androgen
    - inhibin

3. *actions*
   male
   - enhances testosterone secretion (Leydig cell responsiveness to LH)
   - stimulates spermatogenesis
   female
   - stimulates follicle development (see Ch. 8)

## LH (luteinizing hormone)

### Physiology
1. *synthesis* (gonadotroph cell)
   - prohormone unknown
   - glycopeptide, similar to TSH, FSH
2. *control*
   Stimulation:
   - GnRH
   - clomiphene
   Suppression:
   - oestrogen
   - progestin
   - androgen
3. *actions*
   male
   - stimulates testosterone secretion (Leydig cell)
   - stimulates spermatogenesis
   female
   - ovulation (see Ch. 8)

### FSH/LH hypersecretion
- occurs in response to hypogonadism
- relationship to postmenopausal symptoms unclear

### FSH/LH hyposecretion

*Causes*
- hypothalamic
- isolated gonadotrophin deficiency
- pituitary tumours
- panhypopituitarism

*Clinical features*
- hypogonadism (see Ch. 8)

*Investigations*
- hypogonadism (see Ch. 8)
- general pituitary investigations

*Management*
- clomiphene   if appropriate
- GnRH

## POSTERIOR PITUITARY

- Embryologically derived from ventral diencephalon — the neurohypophysis.
- Unmyelinated nerve tracts from paraventricular and supraventricular nuclei terminate onto fenestrated capillaries in the neurohypophysis.
- Hormone synthesis occurs in cell body and transported within carrier protein-neurophysin down axon for secretion into circulation.
- Oxytocin and vasopressin are major secretory hormones of the neurohypophysis
  - both are nonapeptides — differ by 2 amino acids from each other
  - derived from common phylogenetic precursor i.e. vasotocin of lower vertebrates
  - vasopressin predominates in both paraventricular and supraventricular nuclei, but more so in the latter.

### Oxytocin
Stimulation:
- acetylcholine
- angiotensin II
- sexual intercourse
- parturition
- suckling
Suppression:
- catecholamine (via β-receptor)
- stress (via catecholamines)

*Actions*
- Oxytocin may initiate parturition and sustain labour
  - oxytocin is released in increasing spurts by mother, but also by fetus (labour can occur normally in women with oxytocin deficiency)
  - oxytocin receptors on myometrium and parietal decidua are increased during parturition (?oestrogen effect)
  - prostaglandin synthetase in dedidua (but not in myometrium) is stimulated by oxytocin. Prostaglandins cause myometrium contraction and may aid in cervical ripening
  - oxytocin stimulates uterine contractions
- During suckling — oxytocin causes contraction of myoepithelial cells and is essential for the expulsion of breast milk
  - pain or fright inhibits the suckling reflex

### ADH (arginine-vasopressin)

- Octapeptide synthesized in supraoptic and paraventricular nuclei
- Transported down axons for storage in posterior pituitary

### Physiological control
- Plasma osmolality
  - ADH secretion closely linked to osmoreceptor and thirst mechanisms in anterior hypothalamus
  - ADH secretion increases as plasma osmolality rises
  - 1 mOsmol/kg change in plasma osmolality causes a 100 mOsmol change in urine
- ECF volume
  - 'stretch' receptors in thorax and left atrium transmit to hypothalamus
  - 7–15% depletion of plasma volume causes large increase in ADH secretion

### Causes of increased ADH production

*Pituitary origin*
*Cerebral causes*
trauma or surgery
haemorrhage
meningitis, especially tuberculous
encephalitis

- Guillan-Barre-Landry Syndrome
- Cortisol deficiency
- Hypothyroidism
- Congestive cardiac failure
- Positive pressure ventilation
- Hypoglycaemic/emotional stress

*Drugs*
- nicotine
- vincristine
- clofibrate
- barbiturates
- cholinergics

*Ectopic ADH production*
- Carcinoma
- bronchial (oat cell)
- pancreas
- duodenum
- ureter
- bronchial carcinoid
- pulmonary infections — especially TB (from lung)
- Hodgkins disease

# 3. Diseases of the thyroid gland

## PHYSIOLOGY

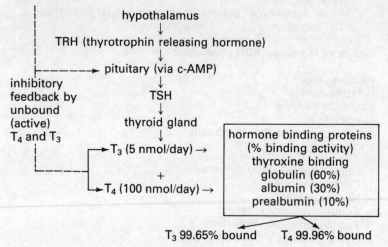

```
                        hypothalamus
                             ↓
        TRH (thyrotrophin releasing hormone)
                             ↓
  ┌ ─ ─ ─ ─ ─→  pituitary (via c-AMP)
inhibitory                   ↓
feedback by                 TSH
unbound                      ↓
(active)              thyroid gland
T₄ and T₃                    ↓
  │              ┌──→ T₃ (5 nmol/day) →
  └ ─ ─ ─ ─ ─ ─ ┤           +
                 └──→ T₄ (100 nmol/day) →
```

hormone binding proteins
(% binding activity)
thyroxine binding
globulin (60%)
albumin (30%)
prealbumin (10%)

$T_3$ 99.65% bound        $T_4$ 99.96% bound

## Thyroid hormone synthesis

TSH — via c-AMP — stimulates thyroid hormone synthesis and secretion pathways.
- increased active uptake of inorganic iodide ($I^-$) by thyroid cells (dietary $I^-$ — 150–1000 $\mu$g/day)
- $I^-$ rapidly oxidized to $10^-$ by peroxidase
- iodination of tyrosine residues on thyroglobulin → monoiodotyrosine (MIT) and di-iodotyrosine (DIT)
- on thyroglobulin molecule, intra-molecular coupling occurs
  DIT + DIT → $T_4$ (major hormone synthesized)
  MIT + DIT → $T_3$ (1/10 synthesis of $T_4$)
- proteolysis of thyroglobin liberates $T_4$, $T_3$ and iodinated tyrosine residues
- $T_4$, $T_3$ to a lesser extent, thyroglobulin and MIT and DIT are secreted into circulation

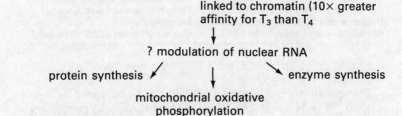

Fig. 3.1

- dehydrogenases remove $I^-$ from tyrosine residues; $I^-$ may be re-used or secreted
- hormones on thyroglobulin molecules are stored in colloid

Peripheral conversion of $T_4$ (Fig. 3.1)

## MECHANISM OF HORMONE ACTION

$T_4$ is converted to $T_3$ and $r\text{-}T_3$ in peripheral tissues and pituitary gland
- Peripheral conversion of $T_4$ is the major source of $T_3$
- $T_3$ is active hormone with $3\times$ metabolic activity of $T_4$
- $r\text{-}T_3$ is inactive hormone with 1/100th the potency of $T_3$

- $T_3 \rightarrow$ avid cellular uptake $\longrightarrow$ intranuclear protein receptor linked to chromatin ($10\times$ greater affinity for $T_3$ than $T_4$

? modulation of nuclear RNA

protein synthesis ↙          ↓          ↘ enzyme synthesis

mitochondrial oxidative phosphorylation

- persistance of protein receptor complex may explain prolonged biological effects of thyroid hormone
- intra-pituitary conversion of $T_4$ to $T_3$ may be mechanism of inhibitory feedback control on release of TSH

**Causes of impaired $T_4$ conversion to $T_3$**
- fetus and newborn
- elderly
- caloric restriction
- hepatic and renal disease
- systemic illnesses and malignancies
- drugs
  - propylthiouracil
  - dexamethasone
  - propranolol
  - amiodarone
  - radiocontrast medium

In many of the above conditions, r-$T_3$ may be elevated and $T_3$ may be low, but the pituitary response to intravenous TRH is normal, and a clinically euthyroid state is present.

## INVESTIGATION OF THYROID DISEASE

- serum $T_4$ and $T_3$ measurements reflect TOTAL (bound and free) hormone content, which parallels changes in thyroid binding proteins — especially thyroxine binding globulin (TBG), FREE (active) hormone concentration re-equilibrates to euthyroid range, despite changes in binding protein concentrations.
- high serum $T_4$ (though with normal $T_3$ and free $T_4$) can occur in familial hyperthyroxinaemia (autosomal dominant) due to an abnormal 'albumin like' protein which binds $T_3$ and $T_4$.

| ↑ Hepatic synthesis of TBG (i.e. elevates $T_4$) | ↓ TBG (i.e. lowers $T_4$) |
|---|---|
| Pregnancy and oestrogens | Testosterone |
| Myxoedema | Thyrotoxicosis |
| Clofibrate and phenothiazines | Corticosteroids and Cushings |
| Acute intermittant porphyria | Protein loss and catabolism |
| Hepatitis and chronic liver disease | Acromegaly |
| Genetic X-linked (increased TBG) | Genetic X-linked (TBG decreased) |

- certain drugs displace $T_4$ from TBG (i.e. cause 'low' $T_4$) eg. salicylate and phenytoin.
- changes in thyroid hormone binding can be assessed by in-vitro $^{125}I$ — $T_3$ binding as in resin uptake studies. By combining this with total serum $T_4$, free thyroxine index can be calculated, which correlates with 'free' active hormone concentrations.
  i.e. free thyroxine index (FTI)
  $$= \frac{\text{serum } T_4 \text{ (or equivalent formulae)}}{T_3 \text{ resin uptake}}$$

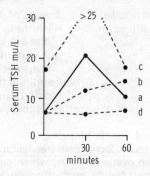

**Fig. 3.2**

- free hormone levels can be measured but technique is not widely available.
- serum TSH — normally low, but useful in hypothyroidism diagnosis and treatment.
- TRH (throtrophin-releasing hormone) 200 μg i.v. with serial TSH measurement at 20 and 60 minutes (Fig. 3.2).
    a. normal response or hypothalamic response
    b. classical hypothalamic response
    c. exaggerated response of hypothyroidism (primary)
    d. flat TSH response occurs in
        - thyrotoxicosis, $T_3$ toxicosis, recently treated toxicosis
        - exopthalmic (euthyroid) Graves — 50%
        - hypopituitary — secondary hypothyroidism
        - Cushing's syndrome and steroids
        - growth hormone
        - iatrogenic or factitious $T_4$ or $T_3$ administration

**Radioactive thyroid scanning**
- $^{131}I$, $^{125}I$, and $^{99m}Tc$ pertechnetate are concentrated in thyroid (and salivary) gland, however, $^{99m}Tc$ is not incorporated into thyroid hormone synthesis. Radiation dose is highest with $^{131}I$, and $^{99m}Tc$ is more commonly used.
- scanning useful in assessing goitre and nodule function. Lesions of 0.5–0.8 cm diameter can be resolved using gamma camera with pin hole collimator i.e. beyond clinical palpation. Radioactive uptake is increased in hyperactive thyroid gland or nodule; a 'hot' nodule is unlikely to be malignant.
- $^{131}I$ is useful in assessing extent of retrosternal goitre extension, as radioactive emission low from other isotopes.

*Causes of enhanced uptake*
Graves disease — diffuse or nodular
Toxic adenoma

*Causes of decreased uptake*
Hashimoto's/atrophic thyroid disease
Subacute thyroiditis — transient
Factitious thyrotoxicosis
Iodide trapping defect
High iodide intake

**Ultrasonography and needle biopsies**
- Ultrasound can detect 2 cm diameter lesions, and differentiates between solid and cystic nodules, which can then be biopsied by needle. In expert hands, such procedures have high diagnostic yield (>90%).

## AUTOIMMUNE THYROID DISEASE

**Pathogenesis (Fig. 3.3)**
- autoimmune thyroid disease (Graves, Hashimoto's, primary myxoedema) 4–8 times commoner in women
- autoantibody and cellular immune activity may determine type of thyroid disease; significance of immune complexes (antibody-thyroglobulin etc.) not known
- thyroid antibodies are probably produced by lymphocytes infiltrating thyroid gland

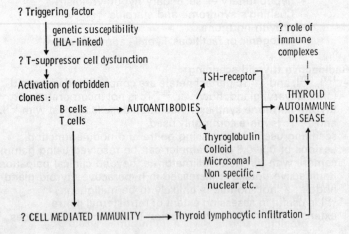

? Triggering factor

genetic susceptibility (HLA-linked)

? T-suppressor cell dysfunction

Activation of forbidden clones :
B cells
T cells → AUTOANTIBODIES

TSH-receptor

Thyroglobulin
Colloid
Microsomal
Non specific -
nuclear etc.

? role of immune complexes

THYROID AUTOIMMUNE DISEASE

? CELL MEDIATED IMMUNITY → Thyroid lymphocytic infiltration

Fig. 3.3

**Table 3.1**

| Disease | HLA association | Receptor antibody | Clinical effects |
|---|---|---|---|
| Graves disease | B8, DRW3 (ethnic variation) | thyroid simulating immunoglobins 70–90% + thyroid growth immunoglobins (? different TSH receptor site) | thyrotoxicosis +goitre (absent in 3–10%) neonatal thyrotoxicosis |
| Graves exophthalmos | | autoantibody to orbital muscle antigen | ? ophthalmic eye disease |
| Hashimotos disease | DR5, DRW3 | TSH-blocking immunoglobins inhibit c-AMP + thyroid growth immunoglobin | hypothyroidism with goitre |
| Atrophic thyroiditis | DR3, B8 | thyroid growth blocking immunoglobin + TSH blocking immunoglobin | hypothyroidism with atrophic gland i.e. primary myxoedema |
| ? Simple goitre | ? | thyroid growth immunoglobins in some cases | euthyroid goitre |

- TSH receptor may have multiple antigenic sites so that autoantibodies to receptor can stimulate or block hormone production or gland growth (see Table 3.1)
- autoantibodies can fluctuate despite medical or surgical intervention, correlating with disease activity
- receptor autoantibodies decrease during pregnancy, but at critical maternal antibody titres, can cross placenta to influence fetal thyroid, e.g. 1% of mothers with past or previous Graves disease can produce thyrotoxic neonate. Transient fetal hypothyroidism can also occur due to passage of thyroid blocking antibodies from the mother

**Use of antibody measurements**
- differential diagnosis of thyroid goitre
- differential diagnosis of unilateral exophthalmos
- ? prediction of relapse of autoimmune thyroid disease
- ? prediction of neonatal Graves disease by estimation of maternal autoantibody titres

## Effects of drug therapy
– Carbimazole and its active metabolite methimazole decrease circulating TSH receptor antibodies in Graves and microsomal antibody in Hashimoto's disease — probably by immunosuppression of lymphocytes in gland

## THYROID GOITRE

### Causes

'PHYSIOLOGICAL' GOITRE
puberty
pregnancy

HYPERTHYROID GOITRE

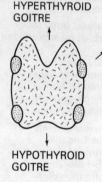

HYPOTHYROID GOITRE

EUTHYROID GOITRE
endemic
sporadic
goitrogens —
foods/drugs
neoplasm
dyshormonogenesis
Riedels thyroiditis
septic (pyogenic) thyroiditis
chronic inflammatory
    TB
    sarcoid
    syphilis

## EUTHYROID GOITRES

### Endemic goitre
– occurrence of goitre in high prevalence area. 200 million people affected in world

*Aetiology (multifactorial)*
iodine deficiency;
goitrogens in water, food inhibit iodine uptake;
mild dyshormono-genesis

→ decreased thyroid hormone synthesis

↓

compensatory chronic TSH stimulation

↓

follicular glandular hyperplasia → goitre ↗ nodular
↘ multinodular (usually irreversible)

*Clinical features*
- spontaneous involution or suppression of follicles results in nodular characteristic
- size of goitre related to duration
- pain in goitre suggests acute haemorrhage
- thoracic inlet compression (rare)
  - dysphagia
  - respiratory problems
  - SVC obstruction

*Investigations*
- $T_4$ (normal or low normal) $T_3$ normal. TSH — usually not elevated
- thyroid scan — [131]I if retrosternal extension present
- thoracic inlet radiology/CT scanning
- single nodules need to be biopsied to exclude malignancy

*Treatment*
- iodine will reverse early follicular hyperplasia
- iodine at later stages may
  - involute follicles and increase nodularity
  - precipitate thyrotoxicosis/$T_3$ toxicosis (Jod-Basedow syndrome)
- routine iodide introduction into population diet has reduced incidence of goitre
- surgery if obstructive goitre present
  - malignancy suspected

**Sporadic goitre**
- occurrence of goitre in area of low prevalence

*Aetiology*
- probably multifactorial — as for endemic goitre. Histopathology similar
- ? autoimmune thyroid disease (thyroid growth immunoglobins)

*Clinical features and investigations*
- 8× commoner in women than in men
- as for endemic goitre

*Treatment*
- iodine ineffective as deficiency likely to be mild
- diffuse goitre reversed with oral $T_4$ suppressive therapy 150 µg per day
- $T_4$ therapy unlikely to be suppressive if thyroid scan shows large number of 'hot' areas as autonomous $T_4$ secretion is likely
- surgery — as for endemic goitre

**Riedels thyroiditis**
- 0.03% of all thyroidectomies. 2–4 times commoner in women. Mean age at diagnosis 50 years

*Aetiology*
- unknown but associated with other idiopathic fibrosing conditions (e.g. retroperitoneal fibrosis, fibrous mediastinitis, sclerosing cholangitis, etc.)
- fibrosis of gland is severe and local structures may be involved e.g. recurrent laryngeal nerve, trachea etc.

*Clinical features*
- slow, asymptomatic gland enlargement — stony hard goitre
- acute enlargement with local pain, tenderness, obstructive symptoms

*Investigations*
- ESR may be elevated
- thyroid hormones normal
- thyroid scan — 'cold areas of fibrosis'
- malignancies will need to be excluded

*Treatment and prognosis*
- self-limiting disease
- surgery for
  - confirmation of diagnosis
  - relief of obstruction
- hypothyroidism — rare, and hypoparathyroidism even rarer

## HYPERTHYROIDISM

**Prevalence**
- 0.2–0.4% of population
- women:men 8:1
- HLA B8 : 2.8× risk of developing Graves disease
- HLA DRW3 : 6× risk

**Commonest causes > 95%**
- Graves disease
- autonomous nodule/multinodular goitre

**Rarely**
- thyroiditis — transient thyrotoxicosis
- iatrogenic or factitious use of thyroid hormones
- iodine ingestion (Jod-Basedow)
- placental hormones
  - human chorionic gonadotrophin shares an $\alpha$ subunit protein with TSH, (hydatidiform mole, choriocarcinoma, seminoma etc)

- ? other placental thyrotrophins
- metastatic thyroid carcinoma
- struma ovarii
- TSH secreting tumour + acromegaly
- excess TRH secretion from hypothalamus

## Metabolic consequences of excess thyroid hormones
- increased mitochondrial and Na-K ATPase activity:
  - ? calorigenic effect
  - increased protein contractile mechanisms
- effect on protein synthesis is complex but overall catabolism predominates
- lipoprotein and lipid metabolism increased
  - decreased serum and tissue triglycerides and cholesterol
  - increased LDL turnover
- enhancement of the effects of other hormone responses e.g. catecholamines, glucagon etc. ? up-regulation of hormone receptors

## Clinical features
- goitre: 95% have goitre; 70% exhibit goitre bruit
- skin and hair:
  - smooth, warm and moist skin
  - heat intolerance, night sweats
  - patchy pigmentation
  - vitiligo
  - pretibial myxoedema (5% — specific for Graves; high receptor antibody titres present)
  - onycholysis (10%)
  - soft and straight hair, alopecia can be temporary unless alopecia totalis occurs
- musculo skeletal:
  - proximal myopathy + muscle atrophy
  - myasthenia <1%
  - hypokalaemic periodic paralysis (occurs mostly in Japanese and Chinese)
  - growth spurt in juveniles
  - demineralization of bone — osteoporosis, hypercalcaemia
  - thyroid acropachy (1% — periosteal bone growth with clubbing occurs in Graves)
- neurological:
  - fatigue or hyperactivity (80%)
  - tremor (95%)
  - enhanced reflexes
  - chorea-athetoid-like movements especially in juveniles
- eyes: see separate section

- cardiovascular:
    - (enhanced catecholamine effects and direct hormone action alter cardiac depolarization and contraction)
    - sinus and atrial arrhythmias
    - systolic hypertension
    - high output cardiac failure
- gastrointestinal:
    - weight loss, despite increased appetite (85%)
    - (occasionally weight gain 2%)
    - gut hypermotility — diarrhoea (20%)
    - fat malabsorption
    - hepatosplenomegaly + variable liver function test abnormalities <10%
    - achlorhydria — 3% have pernicious anaemia
- renal function:
    - increased renal blood flow and glomerular filtration rate
- haematology:
    - relative lymphocytosis
    - normochromic, normocytic anaemia if longstanding disease
- endocrine:
    - menstrual disturbances — commonly oligomenorrhoea
    - fertility controversial ? decreased
    - hirsutism in women
    - hair loss in men
    - impotence and gynaecomastia (? increased oestradiol effect)

**Investigations**
- serum $T_4$ and $T_3$ elevated with undetectable TSH. TSH will be high if toxicosis due to TSH secreting pituitary tumour
- measure 'free' hormone levels or free thyroxine index if drug or other potentially interfering factors present
- thyroid scanning for uptake and detection of a 'hot' nodule
- TRH test if clinical and biochemical tests are equivocal
- thyroid auto-antibodies — useful for confirmation of autoimmune thyroid disease

**Treatment**
Policies vary widely — most consider medical therapy as first choice.
- antithyroid drugs (see Table 3.2)
    - immunosuppressive effect of carbimazole may be useful
    - suitable in young patients with moderate goitre
    - can be used during pregnancy where lowering of antibody titre may be an advantage
Duration of drug therapy:
- usually for 12–18 month course
- ? duration of therapy may influence prognosis

**Table 3.2**

| Drugs | Mechanism | Dose | Adverse effects |
|---|---|---|---|
| Carbimazole<br><br>Methimazole | 1. Carbimazole converts to active methimazole<br>2. Blocks iodine binding to hormone precursors<br>3. Decreases thyroid autoantibody levels | 30–60 mg/day in 3 doses for 2–4 weeks then reduce to maintenance 5–15 mg/day. Clinical benefit observed 3–4 weeks after starting drugs | Unpredictable but occur in first 8 weeks — gastrointestinal upset, rashes, reversible marrow depression. Aplasia cutis in neonates. Crosses placenta; breast feeding contra-indicated |
| Propylthiouracil<br><br>Methylthiouracil | 1. Blocks iodine binding to hormone precursors<br>2. Diverts $T_4$ conversion to r-$T_3$ peripherally | 200–300 mg/day in 3 doses for 2–4 weeks, reduce to 50–150 mg/day | As for carbimazole but adverse reactions more frequent with methyl-thiouracil. Breast feeding probably permissible |
| Potassium perchlorate | Competitively inhibits iodide uptake by thyroid gland | 800–1000 mg/day in 3 or 4 doses for 2–4 weeks, reduce to 300 mg/day | Common if 1000 mg/day taken. Fatal aplastic anaemia, hypersensitivity, nephrotic syndrome |
| Propranolol | 1. Antagonizes sympathomimetic effects of thyroid hormones<br>2. Diverts $T_4$ to r-$T_3$ synthesis (minor) | 40 mg 8-hourly. Not recommended as sole therapy. Useful in thyroid crisis | As with β-blockers, small amounts excreted in breast milk |
| $^{131}$Iodine | Interstitial thyroid irradiation destroys cells. | Wide variability — according to mass and activity of gland. 1–8 mCi — single or multiple doses | Hypothyroidism 30–70% during 10–20 year follow up. Contra-indicated in pregnant and young |

– 3–4 monthly monitoring of clinical and biochemical progress
50% will relapse after medical therapy; relapse is associated with:
– no gland shrinkage with therapy
– failure to suppress radioactive isotope uptake by thyroid gland
  after oral $T_3$
– thyroglobulin titres remain elevated during therapy
– ? patients with high autoantibody titres pre-treatment and HLA
  DRW3 or B8 have high relapse rates
$^{131}$I (see Table 3.2) specific indications:
– elderly
– toxic nodule — selectively destroyed
– recurrence of toxicosis after surgery

**Surgery**
– some consider surgery as treatment of choice for
  thyrotoxicosis — subtotal thyroidectomy is usual operation
Preoperative preparation:
– it is essential to establish an euthyroid state to avoid thyroid
  'crisis'
– antithyroid drugs started at least 2 months pre-op
– oral iodine 1–2 weeks pre-op decreases gland vascularity
If patient intolerant of anti-thyroid drugs:
– 40–60 mg propranolol orally 6 hourly — continue up to 6 hours
  pre-op and give i.v. Propranolol 1–2 mg hourly to keep pulse
  <80
– continue drugs postoperatively until euthyroidism established

*Specific indications for surgery*
– relapse after medical therapy
– anticipated poor compliance with drugs or difficult follow up
– drug intolerance
– thoracic inlet compression by goitre
– suspected malignancy
– cosmetic

*Endocrine complications of thyroidectomy*
Early:
– transient tetany 24–36 hrs post-op. $R_x$ oral or i.v. calcium viz.
  30–60 ml of 10% calcium gluconate in 1 litre 5% dextrose —
  infuse to maintain calcium in low-normal range
– thyroid crisis
Late:
– recurrence of thyrotoxicosis 3–8% — can occur > 5 years post-
  operatively
– permanent hypoparathyroidism 2–4% — $R_x$: vitamin D
  metabolites
– hypothyroidism — usually permanent if present 6–12 months
  post-op; incidence increases with duration of follow up — (40%
  at 1 yr and 1% per year thereafter)

*Follow up of hyperthyroid patients*
- clinical and biochemical effects of treatment
- spontaneous relapses and remissions, long term consequences
  of treatment require life-long observations

## EXOPHTHALMIC GRAVES DISEASE

10% of patients are euthyroid.

50–90% of thyrotoxics have eye disease; CT scanning reveals
high incidence of subclinical orbital muscle hypertrophy.

2% of thyrotoxics have severe eye manifestations ('malignant'
exophthalmos).

### Pathogenesis
- lid lag and lid retraction are partly due to increased
  sympathetic tone in levator palpebrae
- infiltrative exophthalmos involves cellular and humoral
  immunity associated with pre-tibial myxoedema, thyroid
  acropachy and high thyroid autoantibody titres
- antibodies to antigen derived from orbital muscles has been
  demonstrated in 74% of patients with exophthalmos and none
  without exophthalmos (Fig. 3.4)

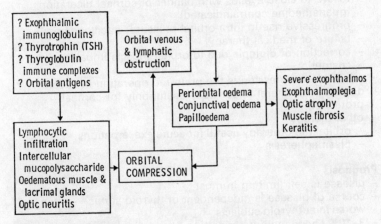

**Fig. 3.4**

### Clinical features
- mild disease
  - stare
  - lid lag and retraction
  - moderate exophthalmos

- severe disease
  - diplopia (worst on upward gaze)
  - photophobia
  - chemosis
  - failure to close eyelid
  - panophthalmitis
  - optic nerve compression
  - corneal ulceration leading to blindness

## Investigations
- exclude other causes of exophthalmos if diagnosis doubtful
- thyroid function tests, orbital autoantibodies
- orbital tomograms
- ultrasonography
- computerized tomography (CT)

## Treatment
- majority will never require treatment; mild disease cosmetically improved with guanethidine eye drops and diuretics. Periobital oedema alleviated by sleeping upright
- severe disease: Prednisolone 60–120 mg per day + azathioprine/cyclophosphamide
- surgical indications:
  - failure to close eyelids with danger of corneal ulceration (guanethedine contraindicated)
  - progressive rise in intra-orbital pressure; papilloedema
  - failure of medical therapy
  - correction of diplopia due to orbital muscle imbalance
  - cosmetic
- orbital decompression is the preferred operation in severe disease with lateral tarsorraphy useful only for corneal protection
- other therapy:
  - orbital radiotherapy useful for acute exacerbations
  - plasmapheresis

## Prognosis
- disease is self limiting in most
- course of disease is independent of thyroid status — often worse in euthyroid subjects
- 3–10% show some deterioration in eye disease when treatment of thyrotoxicosis is initiated and especially if hypothyroidism induced — deterioration may be related to release of thyroid antigens especially thyroglobulins

## THYROID CRISIS
Potentially fatal disorder of increased thyroid hormone action.

**Clinical features**
- high fever
- tachycardia, arrhythmia
- shock, cardiac failure
- diarrhoea, abdominal pain
- jaundice
- hypomania, psychosis
- coma

*Precipitating factors*
- inadequate treatment of severe thyrotoxicosis
- stress — surgical, infection, diabetic ketoacidosis

**Investigations**
- usually very high serum $T_4$ (wide range)

**General measures**
- treat precipitating factors
- tepid sponging, cooling blankets
- hydration

**Specific treatment**
1. Oral anti-thyroid drugs via nasogastric tube — inhibit further hormone synthesis
   - carbimazole 80–120 mg per day *or*
   - propylthiouraul 800–1200 mg per day may be preferred because of peripheral inhibition of $T_4$ conversion to $T_3$.
2. Iodide — 1–2 hours *after* antithyroid drugs stored hormone
   - 1–2 drops of Lugols iodine 8 hourly orally or sodium iodide 0.5–1.0 g i.v.
3. Propranolol inhibits adrenergic component and peripheral $T_4$ conversion:
   - 40–80 mg 4 hourly orally ⎫ monitor pulse rate, blood pressure
   - 2–5 mg 2–4 hourly i.v. ⎭ may precipitate CCF.
4. Steroids — ? prevent cortisol insufficiency ? inhibit peripheral conversion of $T_4$
   - though recommended, overall benefit doubtful
   - hydrocortisone 100 mg 6 hourly i.v.

**Other treatment**
- plasmapheresis and peritoneal dialysis — effectively removes thyroid binding proteins and therefore lowers serum hormones with rapid clinical benefit

# T₃ TOXICOSIS

3–10% of thyrotoxicosis patients; incidence higher in iodine deficient areas.

## Causes
- early phase of diffuse goitre toxicity
- hot nodule
- tri-iodothyronine ingestion
- ? iodine administration to patients with iodine deficiency

## Investigations
- serum $T_3$ elevated, serum $T_4$ normal
- TRH test — flat TSH response
- isotope scanning may
  - reveal 'hot' nodule
  - be suppressed suggesting triiodothyronine ingestion

## Treatment
- as for thyrotoxicosis, and nodules

# HYPOTHYROIDISM

## Prevalence
- spontaneous hypothyroidism
  - 0.01 to 0.08% of population
  - 1/10th frequency of toxicosis
  - maximal incidence in women (80%) and at 30–60 years of age

## Primary gland failure
Commonly (>90%)
- autoimmune thyroiditis (Hashimoto's disease; idiopathic atrophy)
- gland destruction (radioiodine, surgery)
Rarely
- subacute thyroiditis
- gland dysgenesis
- inherited abnormalities of thyroid hormone synthesis:
  - iodide trapping defect
  - peroxidase defect
  - dehalogenase defect
  - coupling defect
  - thyroglobulin synthesis defect

- secondary infiltrations:
  - lymphoma and metastatic carcinoma
  - sarcoidosis
  - amyloidosis
  - cystinosis
- drugs:
  - monovalent anions (iodide, perchlorate, thiocyanate, nitrate)
  - anti-thyroid drugs, sulphonylureas
  - PAS, phenylbutazone
  - lithium
  - cobalt
  - resorcinol
  - cholestyramine

## Secondary hypothyroidism (<5%)
- pituitary disease or tumour
- isolated TSH deficiency
- hypothalamic disease or tumour
- isolated TRH deficiency
- peripheral unresponsiveness to thyroid hormones
  (? nuclear receptor deficiency — familial)

## Metabolic consequences of thyroid hormone deficiency
- ATP utilization reduced causing dysfunction of:
  - thermogenesis with reduced $O_2$ consumption
  - muscle contraction
  - secretory mechanisms e.g. sweat glands
  - Na–K exchange (increased red cell $Na^+$)
- Protein synthesis decreased: growth retardation, neurological retardation
- Lipoprotein metabolism and lipolysis decreased:
  - hypercholesterolaemia (80%)
  - increased fat storage
  - increased LDL (reduced turnover)
- Abnormal connective tissue metabolism:
  - mucopolysaccharide, hyaluronic acid accumulation in skin, conjunctiva and joints
  - protein rich serous infusions in pleura, pericardium and synovium

## Clinical features (due to above)
- Skin and hair
  - dry, flaking skin + carotenaemia tint (85%)
  - puffiness of hands, eyes and face
  - hair loss, alopecia (50%)
  - cold intolerance (80%)

- Musculo skeletal:
  - muscle bulk increased, glossomegaly (20%), vocal chords — hoarseness (60%)
  - muscle cramps, stiffness, paramyotonia
  - muscle enzymes CPK, SGOT, LDH are all elevated
  - arthralgia and synovial effusions
  - osteoporosis
  - retarded skeletal growth in young — bone age lags behind chronological age
  - alkaline phosphate levels are reduced
- Neurological:
  - lethargy and slowed mentation (80%) — reduced cerebral blood flow.
  - fits, coma, dementia, psychosis
  - ataxia (cerebellar involvement)
  - nerve entrapment (Carpal tunnel, rarely VII nerve palsy) (50%)
  - perceptive deafness (40%); defective taste and smell (80%)
- Cardio-respiratory:
  - bradycardia (14%)
  - reduced cardiac output, cardiac failure very rare
  - pericardial effusion (small, tamponade very rare)
  - cardiomyopathy with ECG changes — T wave flattening or inversion
  - ischaemic heart disease
  - hypoventilation
  - pleural effusion
- Gastrointestinal:
  - constipation (50%)
  - obstruction of intestine and peritoneal effusions are rare
  - achlorhydria; gastric parietal cell antibody occur in 30%; pernicious anaemia in 12%
- Renal function:
  - reduced renal blood flow and glomerular filtration rate causes elevation of urea and creatinine
  - water retention, (but plasma volume reduced)
  - hypocalcaemia (rare)
- Haematology:
  - normochromic normocytic anaemia occurs in 50%
  - microcytic or macrocytic anaemias also occur
  - pernicious anaemia in 12%
  - minor coagulation defects, factor VIII reduced
- Endocrine:
  - menstrual disturbance: menorrhagia; amenorrhoea and galactorrhoea with hyperprolactinaemia can occur
  - impaired fertility — (controversial)
  - impaired growth hormone and ACTH pituitary response to insulin induced hypoglycaemia

- impaired cortisol synthesis, but cortisol clearance reduced
- autoimmune adrenal gland insufficiency may be present
- Drugs:
  - metabolism of many drugs impaired, e.g. digoxin, cortisol —
    Cushings syndrome can occur at sub-optimal replacement
    doses of steroids

## Investigations
- serum $T_4$ and $T_3$ are low
- TSH elevated in primary hypothyroidism
- TSH low in secondary hypothyroidism
  - pituitary failure: flat TSH response to TRH
  - hypothalamic disease: TSH increases with TRH
- high titres of thyroid autoantibodies in >80%

## Treatment
- L-thyroxine is used; no advantage in using triiodothyronine
- 90% will eventually be maintained on 150–200 μg L-thyroxine
- rapid restoration of euthyroidism may be hazardous, start with
  dose of 25–50 μg L-thyroxine with increments of 25–50 μg at
  2–4 week intervals
- earliest clinical response is weight loss due to diuresis
- TSH will fall and stabilize after 4–8 weeks at a given dose
- pericardial effusion can take 9 months to resolve

## Ischaemic heart disease and hypothyroidism
- low doses of 25 μg L-thyroxine should be used and increases
  made after clinical assessment of cardiac status, including ECG.
  Increase by 25 μg L-thyroxine every 2–3 weeks. Increased
  severity or frequency of angina attacks should guide
  replacement dose
- long acting nitrites, or propranolol can be used — latter contraindicated in heart failure
- gradual replacement should also be used in heart failure which
  may be exacerbated if replacement too rapid
- dose of digoxin may need to be decreased as sensitivity is
  increased during thyroid hormone replacement

## Adrenal insufficiency and hypothyroidism
- increased rate of metabolism may precipitate Addisonian crisis
  due to:
  - hypopituitarism (especially hazardous)
  - associated autoimmune adrenal disease
  - slower recovery of previously suppressed pituitary-adrenal
    axis
- if hypothyroidism known to be secondary to hypopituitarism
  steroids should be started with thyroxine

## Myxoedema coma
- end-stage of undiagnosed hypothyroidism characterized by
  - hypothermia, bradycardia, myxoedematous features
  - hypoglycaemia
  - hypoventilation with respiratory acidosis and $CO_2$ narcosis
  - excess ADH with hyponatraemia
  - elevated serum lactate, creatine phosphokinase
  - progressive stupor, hypotension and death
- therapy
  - 100 mg hydrocortisone succinate 6 hourly (adrenocortical insufficiency may occur)
  - 500 $\mu$g L-thyroxine intravenously or via nasogastric tube
  - clinical improvement 6–36 hours — if not, consider other cause for coma
  - underlying infection should be treated if present
- prognosis: 80% survival rate

## Subclinical hypothyroidism
- asymptomatic individuals may have normal or low normal serum thyroid hormones and high TSH which maintains near normal euthyroid hormone output
- TSH concentration alone has not predictive value, but if there are high titres of thyroid auto-antibodies then approximately 3–5% may develop hypothyroidism per annum
- annual checks on thyroid function or start L-thyroxine if follow-up not feasible

## Inherited abnormalities of hormone synthesis
- commonest are probably iodide organic binding defects e.g. peroxidase defects
- usually familial — autosomal recessive inheritance
- heterozygotes may have very mild abnormalities
- severity of enzyme defects determines clinical presentation:
  - severe disease present as sporadic goitrous cretinism
  - mild disease present with later onset of goitre and adult hypothyroidism
- iodide organic binding defect can be associated with nerve deafness of varying severity (Pendreds syndrome)
- malignant change may occur in goitre

*Treatment*
- most will require $T_4$ to achieve euthyroidism and suppress TSH induced goitres. Children born to affected families should be screened for myoedema as early as possible

**Subacute thyroiditis (de Quervain, granulomatous, giant cell)**
Viral aetiology likely:
- can occur after virus infections
- geographical and seasonal clustering
- mumps, enteroviruses, influenza, adenovirus may be implicated
Clinical features:
- thyroid pain — acute onset + radiation to ear or jaw;
  dysphagia, hoarseness
- fever lassitude — can be extreme
- tender goitre with overlying erythema
Investigations:
- ESR elevated
- acute phase may show biochemical toxicosis with low radioisotope uptake
- autoantibodies, as in Hashimoto's, can occur transiently or
  rarely persist (mainly thyroglobulin antibody)
Therapy:
- aspirin analgesia usually suffices
- severe, persistant pain dramatically responds to prednisolone
  30–40 mg/day
Prognosis:
- no treatment shown to influence course of disease
- symptoms may persist for months
- permanent hypothyroidism with persistent auto-antibody is a
  rare sequel

*Other causes of pain in gland*
- haemorrhage into thyroid cyst (commonest)
- malignancy
- pyogenic/tuberculous infections
- autoimmune thyroid disease (occasionally)

**Post partum (transient) thyroid dysfunction**
- Subclinical autoimmune thyroid disease has been estimated to
  be as high as 8.5% in women (Japan). Immunological effect of
  pregnancy is to suppress thyroid autoantibody levels which
  may 'rebound' post-partum to higher levels before declining
  back to pre-pregnancy levels. This mechanism may explain
  why 5.5% of post-partum women (Japan) have transient
  thyroid abnormalities
- During 'rebound' phase, a woman may become clinically
  hypothyroid or hyperthyroid depending on her autoantibody
  profile. Dysfunction usually occurs 3–5 months post partum
  and then remits at 5–10 months
- Women most at risk are:
  - those with goitre which persists or enlarges post partum
  - those who gave birth to a girl
  - high thyroid autoantibody titres
- In some women thyroid dysfunction may persist

**Table 3.3**

| Pathology (frequency %) | Average age | Histology | Comments | Treatment | Prognosis |
|---|---|---|---|---|---|
| Papillary (50–80) | 40 | Well differentiated fronds of cells. Microscopic to large invasive tumours. Multicentric 8–20% | Commonest variety in children. 90% lymph node involvement. I[131] uptake by metastases | If localized <1 cm diameter, partial thyroidectomy. Otherwise, radical thyroidectomy + [131]I + thyroxine to suppress TSH stimulation of malignant cells. | Better in those <40 years with small non-invasive tumours. [131]I uptake by metastatic sites improves prognosis. Overall 83% 5 year survival. |
| Follicular (8–25) | 40 | Well differentiated follicles tending to invade blood vessels. Mixed papillary and follicular can occur. | Early spread by blood — 3% distant metastases. 10% local lymph nodes. Metastases take up [131]I in 46%. | Radical thyroidectomy [131]I + thyroxine. (High and frequent [131]I doses are associated with leukaemia.) | Overall 65% 5 year survival. |
| Anaplastic (2–10) | 60 | Undifferentiated, variable cell size. | Large cell carcinoma highly invasive; local and distant metastases. | Palliative surgery only. External irradiation preferred. | Small cell: 20–25% 5 year survival. Large cell: <1% 3 year survival. |
| Medullary (7) | 50 | Parafollicular 'C' cell carcinoma; amyloid in stroma. | Familial (autosomal dominant). Secretes calcitonin, ACTH etc. Associated with MEN II, III. 50% local lymph node spread. | Radical excision. (Familial is bilateral.) X-ray resistant. | 50% 5 year survival. |
| Lymphoma (1) | 60 | Variable, can be primary or secondary. Reticulum cell. | Clinically indistinguishable from anaplastic type. ? Multifocal. | Palliative surgery. External irradiation ± chemotherapy. | 50% 2 year survival. 10% 5 year survival. |

## THYROID MALIGNANCY

13–28% of incidental thyroid autopsy specimens have occult
carcinoma — commonly papillary
Clinical prevalence rare at 2–3 per 100 000.

### Clinical features of malignancy
- previous head and neck irradiation 4–35 years ago
- family history (especially for medullary carcinoma)
- asymptomatic neck mass in 85%; usually hard single nodule
- localized lymphadenopathy
- rapid growth; dysphagia, hoarseness — evidence of local
  invasion

### Investigations
- serum $T_4$ and $T_3$ — usually normal
- serum thyroglobulin elevated in metastatic thyroid disease —
  useful in monitoring disease
- plasma calcitonin markedly elevated in medullary carcinoma
- radioactive isotope scanning — usually 'cold nodule'
- ultrasound — solid lesions, but 1–2% of carcinomas are cystic
- needle biopsy — with ultrasound can detect 92% of carcinomas

### Management of carcinoma types
See Table 3.3.

### Thyroid nodules
- present in 4% of adult population and incidence increases with
  age. Incidence higher in women
- 50% are single nodules
- most nodules have decreased radioisotope uptake (cold) on
  scanning and raise the possibility of carcinoma
- nodules with increased isotope uptake (hot) may preferentially
  secrete $T_3$ and cause $T_3$ toxicosis

*Management*
- exclude carcinoma if nodule is 'cold'
- $^{131}I$ — preferential uptake by hot nodule leaving rest of gland
  intact was considered to reduce risk of hypothyroidism with $^{131}I$
  therapy. In practice $^{131}I$ may fail to eradicate autonomous nodule
  and cause hypothyroidism in about 30%
- surgery — may be preferred — particularly if pathology of
  nodule is uncertain

# 4. Disorders of calcium metabolism

## CALCIUM

### Physiology (Fig. 4.1)

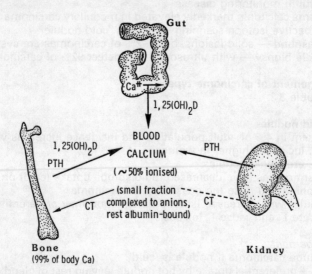

Gut

$Ca^{++}$

$1, 25(OH)_2D$

$1, 25(OH)_2D$

PTH

BLOOD

CALCIUM

PTH

($\sim$50% ionised)

CT

(small fraction
complexed to anions,
rest albumin-bound)

CT

Bone
(99% of body Ca)

Kidney

**Fig. 4.1**

## HYPERCALCAEMIA

### Causes
1. Increased intake — e.g. milk-alkali syndrome
2. Decreased output — e.g. acute renal failure, thiazide diuretics
   (transient)

3. Hormonal disturbance
   a. calcium-regulating hormones
      - hyperparathyroidism
      - hypervitaminosis D
      - sarcoidosis
   b. other hormones
      - hyperthyroidism
      - acromegaly
      - hypoadrenalism
4. Malignancy
   - e.g. carcinomatosis
   - myelomatosis
   - reticuloendothelial disorders
   - local and systemic factors
      - e.g. prostaglandins
      - osteoclast activating factor (OAF)
      - ectopic PTH secretion (rare)
5. Increased bone calcium mobilization
   - immobilization in high bone turnover states e.g. Paget's disease
6. Drugs
   - e.g. vitamin D metabolites and analogues
7. Other
   - e.g. idiopathic hypercalcaemia of infancy

**Clinical features**
- renal
   - calculi, nephrocalcinosis
   - polyuria, polydipsia
   - tubular disturbances
   - renal failure
- psychiatric
   - depression, anxiety
   - psychosis, neurosis
   - personality change
   - dementia
- gastrointestinal
   - constipation, nausea, vomiting
   - abdominal pains
   - pancreatitis, acute and chronic
   - peptic ulceration
- others
   - hypertension
   - corneal calcification

**Investigations**
- plasma calcium, phosphate, alkaline phosphatase
- hormone measurements
  - e.g. PTH
  - vitamin D metabolites
  - thyroid hormones
- exclude malignancy
  - e.g. chest radiograph
  - bone isotope scan
  - blood film
  - Bence-Jones protein

**Treatment**
- acute
  - rehydration
  - calcitonin/diphosphonate
  - steroids
  - haemodialysis
- chronic
  - low calcium diet
  - treat underlying cause

## HYPOCALCAEMIA

**Causes**
1. Hormonal disturbances
   - hypoparathyroidism
   - pseudohypoparathyroidism
   - vitamin D deficiency
   - chronic renal failure
   - magnesium depletion
   - vitamin D dependent rickets types I and II
2. 'Shock' syndromes
   - e.g. acute pancreatitis
   - septicaemia
3. Malignancy
   - e.g. prostatic carcinomatosis
4. Drugs
   - e.g. cytotoxic drugs

**Clinical features**
- tetany
  - carpopedal spasm
  - laryngeal stridor
  - paraesthesia
  - latent (Chvostek's, Trousseau's signs)

- epilepsy
- psychosis
- cataract formation (interferes with lens metabolism)
- basal ganglion calcification — may have extrapyramidal abnormalities
- chronic candidiasis — poor skin health
- skeletal — e.g. rickets and osteomalacia

**Investigations**
- plasma calcium, phosphate, magnesium
- hormonal measurements
  - e.g. PTH
  - vitamin D metabolites
- radiology
  - e.g. skeletal X-rays

**Treatment**
- acute
  - intravenous calcium
- chronic
  - treat underlying cause
  - oral calcium supplements
  - vitamin D metabolites

**PTH (parathyrin)**

**Physiology**
1. *Synthesis* (parathyroid cells) (Fig. 4.2)
   - intact hormone (mainly) + fragments secreted by gland
   - major peripheral cleavage in liver (Kupfer cells)
   - clearance by kidney
   - N terminal fragment short half-life; C terminal half-life longer

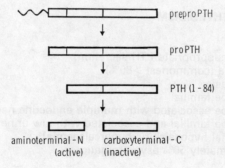

aminoterminal - N    carboxyterminal - C
(active)             (inactive)

**Fig. 4.2**

2. *Control*

$$
\begin{array}{l}
\text{calcium} \uparrow \\
\text{phosphate} \downarrow \\
\text{(magnesium} \uparrow) \\
?\ \ 1,25(OH)_2\,D \uparrow
\end{array}
\ :\ \text{PTH} \downarrow
$$

$$
\begin{array}{l}
\text{calcium} \downarrow \\
\text{phosphate} \uparrow \\
\text{(magnesium} \downarrow)
\end{array}
\ :\ \text{PTH} \uparrow
$$

- severe magnesium depletion interferes with PTH secretion and receptor function
3. *Actions* (Fig. 4.3)

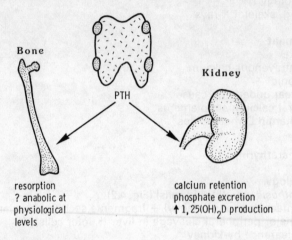

Bone

Kidney

PTH

resorption
? anabolic at
physiological
levels

calcium retention
phosphate excretion
↑ 1, 25(OH)$_2$D production

**Fig. 4.3**

## HYPERPARATHYROIDISM

**Causes**
1. Primary (inappropriate PTH secretion)
   - adenoma (commonest >80%)
   - hyperplasia
     - may be familial
     - may be associated with multiple endocrine neoplasia
     - may be familial and associated with low urine calcium (familial hypocalciuric hypercalcaemia)
   - approximately 50% asymptomatic

2. Secondary (appropriate PTH secretion)
   - chronic renal failure
   - malabsorption
     - gastrointestinal disorders
     - hepatobiliary disorders
   - other causes of hypocalcaemia
3. Tertiary (autonomous PTH secretion superimposed on previous secondary hyperparathyroidism)
   - should be evidence of previous secondary hyperparathyroidism
4. Parathyroid carcinoma
   - extremely rare
   - rapid onset, severe symptoms
5. Ectopic PTH secretion
   - very rare
   - hypernephroma
   - squamous cell lung carcinoma

## Clinical features
Same as hypercalcaemia.
Additionally:
- bone disease
  - osteoporosis
  - osteitis fibrosa cystica
- myopathy
- arthropathy
- associated vitamin D deficiency

## Investigations
- plasma calcium, phosphate
- alkaline phosphatase
- parathyroid hormone assay
- urinary calcium excretion
- radiology e.g. hand X-rays

## Treatment
- surgery — removal of adenoma, hyperplastic glands
- surgery contraindicated:
  - low calcium diet
  - high fluid intake
  - oral phosphate
  - oestrogens (especially postmenopausal)
  - calcitonin/diphosphonate
- secondary hyperparathyroidism:
  - remove underlying cause
  - correct plasma calcium level

# HYPOPARATHYROIDISM

## Causes
1. Idiopathic
   - autoimmune, prematurity
2. Congenital
   - developmental defect
   - occasionally associated with absent thymus and immunological abnormalities (Di George syndrome)
3. Surgical
   - vascular disruption
4. Transient
   - thyroid/parathyroid surgery
   - neonatal e.g. prematurity; maternal hyperparathyroidism
5. Magnesium depletion
   - impairment of PTH secretion
   - impairment of PTH receptor action
6. Pseudohypoparathyroidism (see below)

## Clinical features
Same as hypocalcaemia.

## Investigations
- plasma calcium, phosphate, magnesium
- parathyroid hormone assay
- urinary calcium excretion

## Treatment
- correct plasma calcium level
  - calciferol, dihydrotachysterol
  - 1,25 dihydroxycholecalciferol, 1-α-hydroxycholecalciferol

# PSEUDOHYPOPARATHYROIDISM

End-organ resistance to PTH : receptor or post-receptor abnormality

biochemical features alone —————— mixed —————— somatic features alone (pseudopseudohypoparathyroidism)

## Clinical features
- somatic
  - short stature
  - obesity
  - mental deficiency
  - short 4th/5th metacarpal/metatarsal
  - ectopic bone deposition

- biochemical (mild → severe)
  - as for hypocalcaemia

**Investigations**
- serum calcium, phosphate, magnesium
- parathyroid hormone assay (PTH elevated)
- urinary cAMP responses to exogenous PTH
- radiology e.g. hand X-ray for metacarpal measurement; skull X-ray for basal ganglion calcification

**Treatment**
Treatment for biochemical abnormality:
- correct plasma calcium level
  - oral calcium supplements
  - vitamin D supplements

## 1,25(OH)$_2$D (calcitriol)

**Physiology**
1. *Synthesis* (Fig. 4.4)

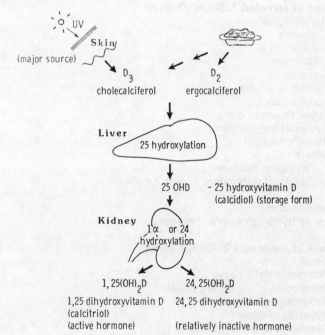

**Fig. 4.4**

2. *Control*
   a. plasma calcium homeostasis

$$\frac{Ca/PO_4}{PTH} \quad \uparrow\downarrow \qquad : \quad 1,25(OH)_2D \quad \downarrow$$

$$\frac{Ca/PO_4}{PTH} \quad \downarrow\uparrow \qquad : \quad 1,25(OH)_2D \quad \uparrow$$

   b. increased calcium need (growth, pregnancy, lactation)

growth hormone
prolactin
placental lactogen        :  $1,25(OH)_2D$  ↑
? oestradiol
calcitonin

   c. variable vitamin D intake (UV light + food)

   250HD                    ↑
24,25(OH)_2D               ↑        :  $1,25(OH)_2D$  ↓
   1,25(OH)_2D             ↑

3. Actions (Fig. 4.5)

## Causes of elevated $1,25(OH)_2D$ levels
1. Physiological
   - growth
   - pregnancy
   - lactation
2. Sarcoidosis
3. Excessive intake
4. Acromegaly
5. Hypocalcaemia per se
6. Hyperparathyroidism
7. Hypothyroidism
8. Others
   - ? hypercortisolism
   - vitamin D dependent rickets type II

*Clinical features*
Same as hypercalcaemia if present.

## Causes of lowered $1.25(OH)_2D$ levels
1. Renal failure
2. Vitamin D deficiency
3. Osteoporosis (postmenopausal)
4. Hypercalcaemia per se
5. Hyperthyroidism
6. Vitamin D dependent rickets type I

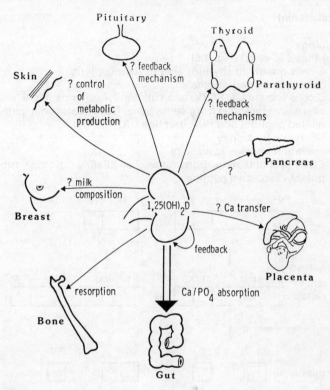

**Fig. 4.5**

7. Others
   – isoniazid therapy
   – ? hypoadrenalism

*Clinical features*
Same as hypocalcaemia and rickets/osteomalacia if present

**Changes in 25OHD levels**
1. Increased
   – excessive intake
2. Decreased
   – vitamin D deficiency
   – antiepileptic therapy
   – antituberculous therapy

## CT (calcitonin)

### Physiology
1. *Synthesis* (C-cells) (Fig. 4.6)
   - C-cells mainly in thyroid; also in thymus, lung, ? parathyroids and adrenals
   - C-cells secrete CT, KC (katacalcin) and ? ? other peptides
   - alternative peptides from same gene, CGRP (calcitonin gene-related peptide) and PDA (peptide DA)
   - clearance by kidney
   - calcitonin species specificity
   - CGRP probable neurotransmitter, ? circulating hormone, most potent vasoactive peptide

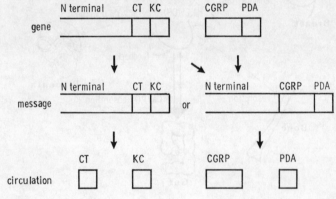

**Fig. 4.6**

2. *Control*
   Stimulation

   | | | |
   |---|---|---|
   | calcium | ↑ | |
   | ? 1,25(OH)₂D | ↑ | |
   | oestrogen | ↑ | |
   | drugs | – pentagastrin | CT ↑ |
   | | – alcohol | |
   | | – glucagon | |
   | | – CCK (cholecystokinin) | |

   Suppression

   | | | |
   |---|---|---|
   | calcium | ↓ | |
   | ovarian hormones | ↓ | CT ↓ |
   | ? corticosteroids | ↑ | |

   - male levels higher than female levels
3. *Actions* (Fig. 4.7)
   - Raised CT levels do not cause hypocalcaemia

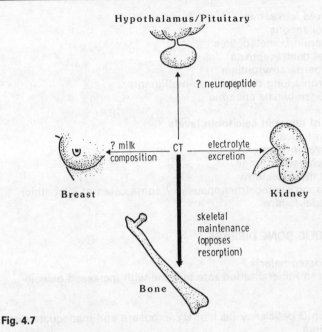

**Fig. 4.7**

## Causes of elevated calcitonin levels
1. Physiological
   - neonates, infants (? growth)
   - pregnancy
   - lactation
2. Medullary thyroid carcinoma
   - sporadic
   - familial
   - multiple endocrine neoplasia type II
     - medullary carcinoma
     - phaeochromocytoma
     - hyperparathyroidism
   - multiple endocrine neoplasia type III
     - medullary carcinoma
     - phaeochromocytoma
     - mucosal neuromas
     - marfanoid habitus
3. Other tumours
   - oat-cell carcinoma
   - breast carcinoma
   - phaeochromocytoma
   - pancreatic endocrine tumours
   - carcinoid tumours

4. Myeloid leukaemia
5. Miscellaneous
   - vitamin D metabolites
   - oral contraceptives
   - hyperparathyroidism
   - chronic lung disease (non-malignant)
   - megaloblastic anaemia

**Causes of lowered calcitonin levels**
1. Physiological
   - lower in women
   - decrease with age
2. Total thyroidectomy
3. Osteoporosis (postmenopausal, ? some cases of idiopathic)
4. Gonadal failure

## METABOLIC BONE DISEASE

**Rickets/osteomalacia**
- impaired mineralization rate in bone with increased osteoid

*Causes*
- vitamin D deficiency (lack of UV exposure and inadequate diet)
  - infants
  - chronic sick, elderly (housebound)
  - Asian immigrants
  - malabsorption syndromes
- impaired hepatic 25-hydroxylation of vitamin D
  - anti-epileptic drugs
  - antituberculous drugs
- impaired renal 1 α-hydroxylation of vitamin D
  - vitamin D dependent rickets type I
  - chronic renal failure
- phosphate depletion, acid-base imbalance
  - renal tubular acidosis
  - vitamin D resistant rickets
  - Fanconi syndrome
- others
  - impaired 1.25 receptor (vitamin D dependent rickets type II)
  - diphosphonate therapy

*Clinical features*
- growing bones — rickets; non-growing bones — osteomalacia
1. Rickets
   - expanded epiphyses
     - wrists
     - knees
     - ankles
     - costochondral junctions (rickety rosary)

- bone deformities
  - bowing of long bones
  - frontal bossing
  - craniotabes
  - open fontanelle
  - expanded sutures
- delayed dentition, enamel hypoplasia
- muscle weakness, hypotonia
- bone pains and tenderness
- symptomatic hypocalcaemia
- family history
2. Osteomalacia
  - bone pains and tenderness
  - proximal myopathy
  - fracture
  - bone deformities
    - bowing of long bones
    - spinal kyphosis
  - symptomatic hypocalcaemia

*Investigations*
- biochemistry

|  | Ca | PO$_4$ | ALP | 25OHD | 1,25(OH)$_2$D |
|---|---|---|---|---|---|
| vit. D deficiency | N or ↓ | N or ↓ | ↑ | ↓ | N or ↓ |
| chronic renal failure | N or ↓ | ↑ | N or ↑ | N or ↓ | ↓↓ |
| vit. D resistance | N or ↓ | ↓↓ | ↑ | N | N or ↓ |
| vit. D dependence type I | ↓ | ↓ | ↑ | N | ↓↓ |
| vit. D dependence type II | ↓ | ↓ | ↑ | N | ↑ |
| tubular acidosis/Fanconi | N or ↓ | ↓ | ↑ | N | N |

- urine calcium usually low
- calcium × phosphate product usually low
- check renal function, acid-base balance, hepatic function, etc.
- radiology
  - expanded metaphyses
  - cupping and irregularity of shaft ends
  - generalized osteopenia
  - biconcave (codfish) vertebrae
  - Looser zone (pseudofracture) — osteomalacia
- bone quantitative histology
  - impaired mineralization (tetracycline labelling)
  - increased osteoid

*Treatment*
- prophylaxis — vitamin D supplements to 'at risk' population
- vitamin D deficiency
  - calciferol (ergocalciferol)
- impaired hepatic 25-hydroxylation
  - 1.25 dihydroxycholecalciferol
- impaired renal 1α-hydroxylation
  - 1,25 dihydroxycholecalciferol
  - 1 alpha hydroxycalciferol
  - dihydrotachesterol
- phosphate depletion
  - phosphate supplements
- acid-base imbalance
  - alkali

Selection of treatment depends on type of disease and biochemical findings.

## Osteoporosis
- reduced bone mass with normal mineralization

*Causes*
- postmenopausal
- age-related (senile)
- endocrine disorders
  - hyperparathyroidism
  - hyperthyroidism
  - hypercortisolism
  - hypogonadism
  - diabetes mellitus
- malignant disorders
  - metastatic carcinoma
  - myeloma
  - reticuloendothelial disorders
- connective tissue disorders
  - osteogenesis imperfecta
  - scurvy
  - ? rheumatoid arthritis
- drugs
  - e.g. heparin
    glucocorticoids
    ethanol
- immobilization/weightlessness
- juvenile
- post-pregnancy
- idiopathic

*Clinical features*
- bone pain — especially spine, weight-bearing bones
- fractures — especially vertebral body, femoral neck, distal forearm
- kyphosis, loss of height etc. with vertebral fractures
- evidence of underlying disorder

*Investigations*
- plain radiology, morphometry
- bone quantitative histology
- specialised techniques
  - peripheral photon absorptiometry
  - spinal dual-photon absorptiometry
  - spinal computed tomography
  - total body calcium (neutron activation analysis)
- appropriate tests for underlying cause

*Treatment*
- correct underlying disorder
- specific therapies (± oral calcium supplementation)
  - oestrogen (postmenopause)
  - anabolic steroids
  - fluoride
  - calcitonin
- additional measures
  - exercise
  - stop smoking
  - balanced diet

**Paget's disease of bone**
- excessive osteoclastic resorption with compensatory increased but disorganised bone formation

*Cause*
- abnormal population of osteoclasts,? slow virus infection
- slight familial tendency
- geographical distribution (disease of Western Europeans)
- affects middle-aged and elderly, both sexes

*Clinical features*
- bone pain in affected site
- pathological fractures
- bone deformities
  - increased skull size, frontal bossing
  - basilar invagination, platybasia
  - bowing of weight-bearing bones
  - increased warmth and tenderness

- neurological complications
  - cranial nerve impairment
  - spinal cord dysfunction
  - cerebellar distortion
  - cerebral steal syndromes
- osteoarthritis
- deafness (per se)
- immobilisation-hypercalcaemia
- increased cardiac output
- sarcomatous change (<1%)

*Investigations*
- biochemistry
  - raised serum alkaline phosphatase
  - raised urinary hydroxyproline excretion
- radiology
  a. osteolytic disease
     - 'v'-shaped resorption fronts
     - cortical resorption clefts
     - ill-defined skull translucencies (osteoporosis circumscripta)
  b. osteosclerotic disease
     - expansion of bone
     - widened cortices
     - loss of trabecular pattern
     - fissure fractures
- isotope bone scanning — defines extent of disease

*Treatment*
- general
  - simple analgesia
  - treatment of concomitant osteoarthritis
  - correction of limb shortening
- indication for specific treatment
  - Pagetic bone pain
  - osteolytic lesions in weight-bearing bones (calcitonin)
  - neurological complications (excluding deafness)
  - immobilization hypercalcaemia
  - major orthopaedic surgery
- specific treatment
  a. calcitonin (extracted porcine, synthetic salmon)
  b. diphosphonate (disodium etidronate)

**Renal bone disease**
- renal osteodystrophy due to parathyroid overactivity and defective mineralisation

*Causes*
- any cause of chronic renal failure (Fig. 4.8)

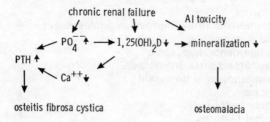

**Fig. 4.8**

*Clinical features*
- bone pain and deformity
- fractures
- myopathy
- tetany
- soft tissue calcification

*Investigations*
- biochemistry (usual)
  - urea/creatinine raised
  - calcium low or normal
  - calcium raised (Aluminium (Al) toxicity, tertiary hyperparathyroidism)
  - alkaline phosphatase raised
  - PTH raised
  - 1,25 $(OH)_2D$ low or undetectable
- radiology
  - e.g. hand X-rays for osteitis fibrosa cystica
  - rarefaction, pseudofractures
  - 'rugger-jersey' spine

*Treatment*
- phosphate binding agents
- calcium and vitamin D metabolites
- occasionally parathyroidectomy (if calcium raised)
- management of renal failure per se

**Other metabolic bone diseases**
1. *Osteogenesis imperfecta*
   - defective collagen
   - severe forms
     - multiple spontaneous fractures
     - death postnatal or early childhood
     - often autosomal recessive

- mild forms
  - osteoporosis (may improve in adolescence)
  - blue sclerae
  - lax ligaments, hypotonia
  - otosclerosis after 3rd decade
  - often autosomal dominant
- diagnosis
  - family history
  - clinical features
  - fibroblast collagenase production (type III: type I ratio may be altered)
  - bone collagen gene abnormalities
2. *Fibrous dysplasia*
  - monostotic or polyostotic
  - often associated with pigmentation
  - occasionally associated with precocious puberty
  - cortex thinned
    - bowing of long bones
    - fractures
  - high bone turnover
  - m:f at least 1:2
  - no specific treatment
3. *Osteopetrosis*
  - severe form
    - anaemia
    - thrombocytopenia
    - fractures
    - onset in infancy
  - mild form
    - later onset
    - occasional fractures
  - diagnosis
    - radiological (dense bones)
  - treatment
    - bone marrow transplant (severe form)

# 5. Disorders of carbohydrate metabolism

## PHYSIOLOGICAL CONTROL OF INSULIN SECRETION

The coordinated secretion of insulin involves several control mechanisms.
Local control of islet cell function:
- Islets of Langerhans comprise:
  - 25% α cells containing glucagon
  - 65% β cells containing insulin
  - 10% δ cells containing somatostatin
  - 5% PP cells containing pancreatic polypeptide

Electron microscopy studies have demonstrated tight intercellular junctions between the various cell types facilitating local hormone interactions.
- insulin and glucagon secretion is inhibited by somatostatin
- glucagon stimulates the secretion of insulin
- insulin inhibits the secretion of glucagon

Autonomic control:
- Hypothalamus controls pancreatic islet cell secretion during cephalic phase of digestion via autonomic nervous system
  - acetylcholine (vagal) stimulates insulin secretion in presence of glucose
  - α-adrenergic (sympathetic) inhibits insulin secretion
  - β-adrenergic stimulates insulin secretion

### Glucose

Glucose is the most important physiological stimulator of insulin secretion.
- Insulin secretion rises when blood glucose > 5 mmol/l (90 mg/100 ml) and is maximal when blood glucose rises to 15 mmol/l (270 mg/100 ml)
- A biphasic release of insulin is seen after a glucose challenge
  - acute secretory phase (minutes) from mobile insulin pool
  - chronic secretory phase (> 1/2 h) — newly synthesized insulin
- Evidence suggests that glucose metabolites in B cells stimulates the Ca-calmodulin dependent contraction of microtubules resulting in exocytosis of insulin granules

Other insulin secretagogues:
- Most require the presence of glucose for stimulation of insulin release
  - fructose, amino acids — especially leucine and arginine; and fatty acids
  - gut hormones — glucagon, secretin, vasoactive intestinal peptide (VIP), gastric inhibitory peptide (GIP), cholecystokinin and bombesin (gut hormones may be part of the entero-insular axis responsible for the greater release of insulin after oral glucose)
  - prostaglandin $E_2$ can inhibit but usually stimulates insulin
  - endorphins, enkephalins

## INSULIN

### Synthesis
The synthesis of insulin is directed by a gene on the short arm of chromosome 11; nearby nucleotide sequence may influence glucose-insulin regulation (Fig. 5.1).

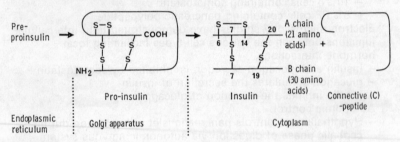

**Fig. 5.1**

PRE-PROINSULIN ⟶ PROINSULIN ⟶ INSULIN (in secretory granules)
endoplasmic reticulum        Golgi apparatus        C-PEPTIDE

Pro-insulin has 5% biological activity of insulin and is converted in equimolar amounts to active insulin and non-active C-peptide. The secretion of C-peptide in plasma is a useful marker of endogenous insulin secretion.

About 60 units per day of insulin are secreted by the normal pancreas.

### Metabolism
Pancreatic insulin ⟶ 50% of insulin removed in single passage through liver ⟶ 30–40% renal degradation ⟶ Peripheral metabolism (fat, muscle etc)

Degradation of insulin occurs by proteolytic enzymes, chiefly in liver and kidney.

Plasma half life of insulin varies with route of injection; absorption is slower and more variable from extravascular sites.

i.v.  – 4 to 5 minutes
i.m.  – 2 hours
s.c.  – 4 hours

*Metabolic effects*

| | | |
|---|---|---|
| Rapid (minutes) | activation of insulin sensitive membrane transport systems (into cell) | – glucose<br>– amino acids<br>– K, Mg, Ca, PO$_4$<br>? fatty acids |
| Gradual (hours) | activation of membrane protein kinase which activates enzymes by ? phosphorylation | – inhibits gluconeogenesis ( ↑ glycogen storage)<br>– inhibits lipolysis ( ↑ fat storage)<br>– ↑ protein synthesis<br>– ↑ DNA/RNA synthesis<br>– ↓ c-AMP (antagonizes effects of hormones that ↑ c-AMP e.g. glucagon, catecholamines, etc.) |

Insulin receptor
– consists of two $\alpha$ and two $\beta$ subunits joined by disulfide bonds, and is similar to somatomedin C (IGF I) receptor
– perturbation of receptor complex may be important in the rapid activation of transport mechanisms by insulin
– protein-kinase closely linked to receptor may initiate the gradual effects of insulin by phosphorylation of key enzymes
– internalization of insulin-receptor complex occurs but importance of this is not known
– 'low' insulin concentration
  – inhibits gluconeogenesis, glycogenolysis, lipolysis
  – stimulates cellular uptake of K
– 'high' insulin concentration
  – stimulates glucose uptake and metabolism

## DIABETES MELLITUS

**Classification** (Table 5.1)

*Insulin dependent diabetes mellitus (Type I)*
1. classical juvenile onset (HLA — DR3/B15 association)
2. associated with polyendocrine abnormalities and organ specific antibodies (HLA — DR3/B8 association)

*Non-insulin dependent diabetes mellitus (Type II)*
– obese/non-obese
Secondary causes
– Pancreatic diseases
– Hypoinsulinaemia
  – hyperaldosteronism
  – somatostatinoma
  – phaeochromocytoma
  – hypocalcaemia
  – hypothalamic defects
– Hyperinsulinaemia (peripheral antagonism of insulin)
  – glucocorticoids (Cushing's syndrome)
  – glucagonoma
  – acromegaly
  – progesterones and oestrogens
– Insulin receptor abnormalities
  – congenital lipodystrophy
  – acanthosis nigricans
  – insulin receptor auto-antibodies
– Abnormal forms of insulin

*Genetic syndromes/associations*
– Inborn errors of metabolism (Glycogen storage Type I; hyperlipidaemia; porphyria)
– Neuromuscular disorders
  – diabetes insipidus, diabetes mellitus, optic atrophy, nerve deafness (DIDMOAD)
  – Friedrich's ataxia
  – Huntington's chorea
  – Laurence-Moon-Biedl
  – muscular dystrophy
– Chromosomal syndromes
  – Down's
  – Turner's
  – Kleinfelter's

**Table 5.1**

|  | Insulin dependent (Type I) | Noninsulin dependent (Type II) |
|---|---|---|
| Aetiology | ? Viral interaction with defective immune response genes (e.g. coxsackie?) Part of familial, polyendocrine autoimmune disease | Peripheral insulin resistance at receptor or postreceptor level: ? Defect of insulin-glucose regulating gene on chromosome 11 |
| HLA associations | HLA-DR3 or HLA-DR4 have 3–5× risk of developing insulin dependent diabetes DR3/DR4 heterozygotes have 20–40× risk (N.B. Ethnic variation) | No known association |
| Auto-antibodies | 60–80% have islet cell antibody (ICA) at diagnosis Declines to 20% after 5 yr Complement fixing ICA may indicate acute phase of disease or antedate onset by several years Organ specific autoantibodies in polyendocrine disease e.g. pituitary antibodies | Incidence as for non-diabetics i.e. <5% |
| Islet pathology | Lymphocyte infiltration and destruction of B cells results in severe insulin deficiency | Normal, or fibrotic or hyaline changes in islets Plasma insulin low or elevated |
| Inheritance | Weak: <10% have family history; 30–50% of identical twins are concordants | Strong: >20% family history and >90% concordance in identical twins |
| Age of onset | Maximal 12–14 years; small peak at 4 years | >30 years |
| Sex | Men > women (slight) | Women > men (gap decreasing) |
| Presentation | Acute (weeks to months) ketoacidosis polyuria polydipsia weight loss | Can be asymptomatic Obesity Acute symptoms may be precipitated by illness or surgery, but ketosis rare Diabetic complications |

*Drugs*
- Diuretics, e.g. thiazides and anti-hypertensive agents, e.g. diazoxide
- Catecholamines/agonists/antagonists
- Pancreatic toxins
  - alloxan, streptozotocin, cytotoxics, nitroso-compounds
- Hormonally active drugs
  - steroids, ACTH, thyroxine (toxic doses)

## Diagnostic and classification criteria
- Classical symptoms with unequivocal hyperglycaemia (plasma glucose >11 mmol/l or 200 mg%)

Fasting hyperglycaemia on more than one occasion:

*Fasting glucose*                     *Action*

venous plasma mmol/l (mg%)
>8 (140) ............................................ Diabetes confirmed
6–8 (108–140) ................................. Do 75 g oral GTT
<6 (108) ............................................ Diabetes excluded

or abnormal glucose tolerance test on more than one occasion:

|  | *Fasting* | *2 h (venous plasma mmol/l)* |
|---|---|---|
| 75 g oral | >8 | >11 diabetic glucose tolerance |
| glucose tolerance | <8 | 8–11 impaired glucose tolerance |

Of those with impaired glucose tolerance, 2–3%/yr progress to diabetes.

Whole blood glucose estimations are 15% lower than corresponding plasma values.

## DIABETIC KETOACIDOSIS

**Causes**
1. Presentation of insulin dependent diabetes mellitus
2. Insulin withdrawal from an insulin dependent diabetic
3. Increased insulin demand during infections, surgery and pregnancy etc.

**Biochemical features (Fig. 5.2)**
- level of hyperglycaemia is not a good guide to severity of acidosis

**Clinical features**

*Early*
- polyuria, polydypsia
- nausea, vomiting
- abdominal pain
- hyperventilation (Kussmaul type)
- dehydration

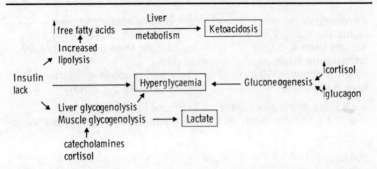

**Fig. 5.2**

*Late*
- drowsiness → unconsciousness
- hypotension → shock
- hypothermia
- death

**Investigations**
- blood glucose
- electrolytes
- urea and creatinine
- arterial pH
- blood count (leucocytosis may be present in absence of infection)
- exclude infections

**Treatment**

*Fluid replacement*
- will vary according to age and weight of patient; central venous pressure catheter is useful in elderly patients or if cardiac disease is present
- use plasma expanders if hypotension present
- N saline (0.9%)
      1 litre over 1/2 h                    – if plasma Na >155 mmol/l,
      1 litre over 1 h × 2                   change to 1/2N saline
      1 litre over 2 h × 2                   (0.45%) if plasma 145–150
      1 litre over 4 h × 2                   then use N saline
      i.e. 7 litre over 14 h                 when glucose < 10 mmol/l, use
      then 1 litre over 6–8 h                dextrose-saline

*Insulin*
- short acting insulin e.g. soluble or actrapid is used. It can be diluted in N/saline for infusion either via a pump, or paediatric drip set

*intravenous regimen*
Bolus i.v. 0.3–0.4 u/kg body
weight then 4–6 u/hr
continuous infusion
when glucose < 10 mmol/l
give 3 u/h

*intramuscular regimen*
Bolus i.m. 0.3–0.4 u/kg body
weight then 5–8 u — hourly
i.m.
when glucose < 10 mmol/l,
give 5–10 u 2 hourly

- glucose should decrease at 3–5 mmol/l/h
- a q.d.s. insulin regimen can be started when patient is able to eat

*Potassium*
- do not give until plasma K known; give as chloride or alternate and monitor frequently

| plasma K (mmol/l) | amount (mmol) to add to 1 L fluid infusions |
|---|---|
| >5 | 0 |
| 4–5 | 20 |
| 3.5–4 | 30 |
| <3.5 | 40 |

*Bicarbonate*
- await plasma pH result; K is given with $HCO_3$

| plasma pH | mmol of $HCO_3$ |
|---|---|
| >7.1 | 0 |
| 7.0–7.1 | 50 + 10 mmol KCl over 30 min |
| <7.0 | 100 + 20 mmol KCl over 60 min |

- Re-check plasma pH after $HCO_3$ infusion and repeat

*Others*
- $O_2$ if arterial $pO_2$ <80 mm Hg (10.6 Kp)
- plasma expanders if BP remains low
- exclude and treat precipitating factors e.g. infections
- phosphate replacement can increase red cell 2, 3 diphosphoglycerate so that $O_2$ dissociates more easily from haemoglobin and theoretically improves tissue oxygenation — doubtful benefit in ketoacidosis
- naso-gastric tube aspiration if unconscious/semiconscious

## Complications of the treatment of diabetic ketoacidosis

*Cerebral oedema*
- ? due to disequilibrium with rapid correction of blood sugar and fluid replacement
- occurrence is difficult to predict, but may be linked to inappropriate use of hypotonic saline (0.45% saline)
- tends to occur in children, and is fatal

*Pulmonary oedema*
- less commonly seen than cerebral oedema though may have similar aetiology
- ? increased pulmonary-capillary permeability

*Hyperchloraemic acidosis*
- due to excessive use of isotonic saline
- characterized by low $HCO_3$ and anion gap, persisting after reversal of ketosis
- usually benign and transient

*Hypoglycaemia*
- rare with low dose insulin therapies
- commoner with high dose insulin protocols

**Prognosis**
Diabetic ketoacidosis is the commonest cause of death in diabetics <20 years of age, and for 16% of all deaths in diabetics under the age of 50 years.
- delay in diagnosis and management contributes to mortality

## HYPEROSMOLAR NON-KETOTIC HYPERGLYCAEMIA

Occurs in non insulin dependent diabetics, characterized by:
- decreased consciousness
- plasma osmolality >330 mmol/l
- arterial pH >7.3 (ketoacidosis absent)
- plasma $HCO_3$ >20 mmol/l

The condition may have been exaggerated by consumption of glucose-containing drinks.

Treatment is similar to that of diabetic ketoacidosis, but if patient is hypotensive use plasma saline initially, switching to hypotonic (0.45%) saline when normotensive.

Mortality is about 10%

## TREATMENT OF INSULIN DEPENDENT DIABETES (Table 5.2)

Highly purified, pork insulins are less antigenic; this may be an advantage.

**Human insulin**
- more rapidly absorbed, quicker onset of action
- allergy can occur but is rare
- useful if allergic to beef or pork insulins or when beef or pork insulin antibodies cause insulin resistance

*Maintenance insulin regimens*
The insulin regimen should be adapted to the requirement of the patient.
- Long or intermediate duration with a short-acting insulin, given twice daily is suitable for young active diabetics. Two-thirds of the total daily insulin requirements may be given before breakfast and the remaining 1/3 before the evening meal. A ratio of 2:1 of long-acting:short acting insulin may be used initially with subsequent changes to dosage according to home monitoring of pre-prandial blood sugar.
- A long acting insulin, e.g. Ultratard given in the morning or evening for basal requirements and short acting insulin, e.g. Actrapid 2–3 times per day half an hour before each meal.
- A single injection of a long acting insulin is suitable for elderly patients, especially if the insulin is to be administered by a district nurse.
- Continuous subcutaneous insulin infusion (CSII). An infusion pump delivers insulin at a constant basal rate with controlled pre-prandial boosts; near-physiological blood sugar control can be obtained. The technique is not without hazard and should only be used under close supervision. Possible indications for CSII are:
  1. Painful diabetic neuropathy
  2. Troublesome hypoglycaemia — though 'brittle' diabetes responds poorly
  3. Pregnancy.

*Complications of CSII*
- hypoglycaemia (pump may continue insulin delivery while patient unconscious)
- pump failure can produce ketosis in a few hours
- infection at site of infusion needle

**Complications with insulin therapy**

*Hypoglycaemia*
- Causes
  - mismatching of insulin regimen to dietary demands
  - exercise — speeds absorption of insulin and lowers blood glucose
  - accidental or deliberate overdose of insulin
  - 'brittle' diabetes
- Hypoglycaemia during sleep may result in rebound morning hyperglycaemia (Somogyi effect). Responds to reduction in evening dose of insulin.

**Table 5.2** Insulin preparations in common use

| Preparation | Onset(h) | Peak effect(h) | Duration(h) | |
|---|---|---|---|---|
| *Short acting* | | | | |
| Soluble BP* | 1 | 3–5 | 8 | |
| Nuso* | 1 | 3–5 | 8 | Beef |
| Neusulin | 1 | 2–6 | 8 | |
| Hypurin neutral | 1 | 2–6 | 8 | |
| Actrapid MC | 1/2 | 3–5 | 7 | Pork |
| Velosulin | 1 | 1–3 | 8 | |
| Human actrapid | 1/2 | 2–5 | 8 | Human |
| Humulin S | 1/2 | 1–3 | 7 | |
| | | | | |
| *Intermediate* | | | | |
| Semilente* | 1 | 4–8 | 16 | Beef |
| Hypurin isophane | 2 | 6–12 | 24 | |
| Semitard MC | 1 | 5–10 | 16 | Pork |
| Insulatard | 2 | 4–12 | 24 | |
| Humulin I | 1 | 2–8 | 20 | Human |
| | | | | |
| *Long* | | | | |
| Lente* | 2 | 6–14 | 29 | |
| Isophane* | 2 | 4–14 | 28 | |
| Hypurin lente | 2 | 8–12 | 30 | Beef |
| Neulente | 2 | 6–12 | 30 | |
| Neuphane | 2 | 6–12 | 30 | |
| Monotard MC | 3 | 6–14 | 22 | Pork |
| Human Monotard | 2 | 7–15 | 22 | Human |
| | | | | |
| *Very long* | | | | |
| Ultralente* | 4 | 10–30 | 36 | |
| Ultratard | 4 | 10–30 | 35 | Beef |
| Protamine* | 4 | 10–20 | 35 | |
| Hypurin protamine zinc | 4 | 10–20 | 35 | |
| | | | | |
| *Biphasic and mixed preparations:* | | | | |
| Mixtard    30% Velosulin | 1 | 2–8 | 24 | |
| 70% Insulatard | | | | Pork |
| Initard    50% Velosulin | 1 | 2–8 | 24 | |
| 50% Insulatard | | | | |
| Rapitard    25% Actrapid MC | 1 | 4–12 | 22 | Beef |
| 75% Crystalline beef | | | | and |
| Lentard MC    30% Amorphous pork | 3 | 7–15 | 24 | pork |
| 70% Crystalline beef | | | | |

Beef insulin differs by 3 amino acids, and pork insulin by 1 amino acid from human insulin.

* not highly purified

- β-blockers retard the sympathomimetic symptoms e.g. tremor, palpitations etc. and prolong the hypoglycaemia. Sweating is not affected.
- Hypoglycaemic coma in a diabetic should be rapidly confirmed, if possible with Dextrostix or BM-Test glycemie 20–800, as exacerbation of a hyperosmolar state or induction of hyperkalaemia with blind intravenous 10–25 g glucose can be avoided. (25 g glucose given intravenously can increase blood glucose by 12 mmol/l).
- 1 mg of glucagon i.m. is useful, as it can be given by non-medical personnel.

*Allergy*
- Indurated erythematous lesion at injection site occurs in up to 1% of diabetics at the start of treatment due to IgE antibodies against insulin or contaminants in insulin preparations (e.g. zinc). The rash resolves spontaneously or with topical steroid therapy.
- Urticaria, angio-oedema and anaphylaxis due to IgG or IgE insulin antibodies are rare, and desensitizing with pork insulin may be required. Pork insulins have also been associated with allergic reactions. Human insulin may avoid such reactions.
- In solution, insulin aggregates due to hydrophobic sites on molecule — these aggregates enhance immunogeneticity and may explain the emergence of antibodies to exogenous human insulin.

*Lipodystrophies*
- lipoatrophy
  - less common with highly purified insulins which can reverse the lesion
- lipohypertrophy
  - occurs at sites of frequent insulin injections and is avoided by rotating injection site

*Insulin resistance*
mild resistance          — 80–125 unit/day
moderate resistance   — 125–200 units/day
severe resistance       — >200 units/day

- Causes:
  mild/moderate
  - obesity
  - surgery, infections, ketoacidosis
  - acromegaly, Cushing's syndrome
  - β-sympathomimetics e.g. salbutamol infusions

severe resistance:
- high titre of IgG insulin antibodies (0.1% of patients) to beef and rarely to pork insulins
- insulin receptor antibodies (Type B insulin resistance) occur
  - with acanthosis nigricans
  - autoimmune disorders
  - IgA deficiency, ataxia telangiectasia
- receptor defects (non-immunological or Type A insulin resistance)
  - acanthosis nigricans
  - lipoatrophic diabetes
  - leprechaunism
  - Rabson-Mendenhall syndrome

*Causes of increased sensitivity to insulin*
- anorexia nervosa
- adrenocortical failure
- hypopituitarism
- 'honeymoon' period at beginning of treatment of insulin dependent diabetes
- changing from beef to pork or human insulins (less binding to insulin antibodies)

*Skin abnormalities with diabetes*
Apart from diabetic dermopathy, none are specific for diabetes. Infections require antibiotics or topical fungal agents, the rest are usually self limiting or require no specific therapy.
*Infections:*
- staphylococcal — boils, carbuncles
- streptococcal — cellulitis
- candidiasis — genitalia, intertriginous areas
- pityriasis versicolor
*Associated with diabetes or impaired glucose tolerance:*
- granuloma annulare
- necrobiosis lipoidica
- diabetic dermopathy
- lichen planus
- acanthosis nigricans (benign, autosomal recessive)
- Werner's syndrome (premature aging of skin, autosomal recessive)
- haemochromatosis
- lipodystrophy
- pemphigoid — localised
- contractural hands (?link with microvascular complications)
*Associated with insulin therapy:*
- local allergic reaction
- fat atrophy
- fat hypertrophy

## Treatment of non-insulin dependent diabetes mellitus

*Diet*
A weight reducing diet is offered if obesity is present. The daily calorie intake should be composed of:
   55% — carbohydrate, preferably as high-fibre, leguminous foods
   25% — fat, half as polyunsaturate
   20% — protein
An initial 1–2 month trial may show that diet alone is sufficient, but start therapy if diabetic control is poor:
– symptoms
– plasma glucose frequently > 10 mmol/l
– glycosylated HbA₁ > 10%

*Oral hypoglycaemics*
Table 5.3 shows some of the available oral hypoglycaemics.

**Table 5.3** Oral hypoglycaemics

| Drug | Plasma half-life (h) | Total dose mg/day | Predominant elimination route |
|------|------|------|------|
| **Sulphonylureas** | | | |
| t.d.s. dose: | | | |
| Tolbutamide | 5–8 | 1000–2000 | hepatic |
| Glipazide | 2–4 | 5–22.5 | hepatic |
| Gliquidone | 2 | 45–180 | hepatic |
| Acetohexamide | 2–5 | 500–750 | renal |
| | | | |
| b.d. dose: | | | |
| Glymidine | 5–8 | 500–1500 | renal |
| Tolazamide | 8 | 100–1000 | renal |
| Glibenclamide | 2 | 5–15 | hepatic |
| | | | |
| o.d. dose: | | | |
| Chlorpropamide | 36 | 250–500 | renal |
| Gliclazide | 12 | 40–320 | hepatic |
| Glibornuride | 8 | 12.5–50 | hepatic |
| **Biguanides** | | | |
| b.d. or t.d.s. dose: | | | |
| Metformin | 3–5 | 1000–2000 | renal |
| Phenformin | 3–5 | | hepatic and renal |

The biological half-life of the drug may be longer due to active metabolites or to the oral formulation.

*Sulphonylureas*
- stimulate insulin release (?via Ca influx into β cells)
- increase insulin receptors (?due to decreased receptor internalization)
- decrease output of glucose from liver
- side effects
  - hypoglycaemia — occurs with long-acting drugs in elderly, and in presence of renal failure; tolbutamide may be used.
  - water retention — associated with chlorpropamide and tolbutamide, both contraindicated in heart failure
  - diuretic effect — with glibenclamide
  - alcohol flushing — inherited autosomal dominant for chlorpropamide (? protects from macro- and microvascular complications)
  - anti-platelet effect — gliclazide (?and glibenclamide) doubtful significance
  - non-specific — gastrointestinal upset, skin rashes, jaundice, leucopenia
  - drug interactions — due to competitive displacement of drug from protein binding sites
  - weight gain — though still used in obese diabetics

*Biguanides*
- mechanism of action controversial
  - enhanced glucose uptake by muscle
  - increased insulin receptors or receptor responsiveness
  - decreased intestinal absorption of glucose
  - inhibition of mitochondrial oxidative phosphorylation (anaerobic metabolism of glucose to lactate occurs)
  - decreased gluconeogenesis

- side effects
  - gastrointestinal upset, anorexia (useful in obese diabetics)
  - lactic acidosis with phenformin (rare with metformin) is associated with 50% mortality — avoid their use in presence of hepatic or renal disease
  - $B_{12}$ malabsorption is a rare complication

**Management of diabetes during surgery**

*Non-insulin dependent diabetes*
Well controlled (plasma glucose persistently < 10 mmol/l)
- omit medication on day of operation
- check plasma glucose post-operatively and then 4 hourly. If plasma glucose > 10 mmol/l — start on subcutaneous insulin (short acting)

Poorly controlled (blood glucose mostly > 10 mmol/l)
- if possible, control diabetes with insulin a few days before operation, and use the intravenous insulin regimens for insulin dependent diabetes

*Insulin dependent diabetes*
Omit usual insulin on the morning of the operation and use the regimens shown:
a. *Variable insulin infusion rate regimen.* Set up 5% dextrose or dextrose-saline infusion at a rate according to the patients fluid requirements, and an insulin infusion system via a Y-connection (pump or paediatric giving set). The rate of insulin infusion is adjusted to maintain blood glucose 4–7 mmol/l.

| Blood glucose (mmol/l) | Insulin rate (u/h) |
|---|---|
| <4.0 | 0–0.5 |
| 4–7 | 1 |
| 7–10 | 2 |
| 10–13 | 3 |
| 13–22 | 4 |
| > 22 | 6 and review |

During and after operation, the plasma glucose is measured hourly, and then 2–4 hourly when plasma glucose is stabilized.

The above insulin infusion rate can be doubled in severely ill patients with increased insulin requirements, and those having cardio-pulmonary bypass procedure where a large intravenous carbohydrate load is administered. Concurrent steroid therapy can double the insulin requirements. Change back to previous regimen, or temporarily use q.d.s. short acting insulin, when patient able to eat.
b. *Insulin-dextrose regimen.* Add 16 u insulin + 10 mmol KCl to 500 ml of 10% dextrose and infuse at 100 ml/h. Check blood glucose 2 hourly:
  >10 mmol/l — change to 20 u insulin
  <4 mmol/l — change to 12 u insulin

**Complications of diabetes**
- Insulin deficiency results in multiple metabolic abnormalities
- Good diabetic control should result in reversal of those metabolic abnormalities that would otherwise result in life-impairing complications
- Complication tend to occur in cells or structures in which glucose transport occurs independent of insulin e.g. nerve cells, capillaries, lens, etc.

*Microvascular disease*
- In diabetes, the earliest microvessel changes are increased thickness and synthesis of basement membrane with increased leakage of plasma.
- Abnormalities of microvessel structure and function may be due to:
  1. Glycosylation of basement membrane proteins during or after synthesis in endothelial cells. May produce a 'porous' basement membrane. This may be the cause of leakage in glomerular capillaries
  2. Endothelial cell dysfunction may allow leakage of plasma in capillaries where basement membrane is intrinsically permeable e.g. retina and brain
  3. Abnormalities of local cells that normally function to clear filtered plasma debris i.e. pericytes in retina and epithelial cells in glomerulus.
- However multiple aetiologies are involved — many are interrelated and most are tenuous (see Fig. 5.3).
- Most constant association with incidence of microvessel disease is duration of diabetes.
- Twin studies suggest genetic susceptibility in NIDDM, but data conflicting in IDDM.

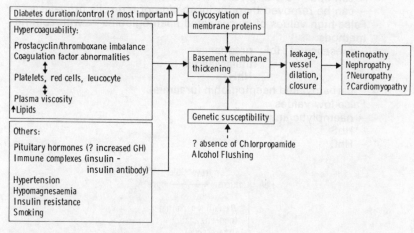

**Fig. 5.3**

*Reversibility of microvascular abnormalities*
- Animal and some human studies suggest that earliest detectable microvascular disease is reversible with strict metabolic control of diabetes. Established microvascular complications are usually irreversible.

- There is wide individual variation in rate of progression of microvascular complications; and in different organ systems — thus proliferative retinopathy may occur in an individual with no clinical evidence of renal disease.
- In general 30% of long surviving diabetics tend to be free of clinical microvessel disease and over 80% are free from incapacitating complications.

## GLYCOSYLATED HAEMOGLOBINS (Fig. 5.4)

- Glycosylated haemoglobin as a percentage of total haemoglobin correlates with degree of glycaemia over preceding 6 weeks
- $HbA_{1c}$ is the major subfraction
- Methods of estimation:
  - column chromatography
  - electrophoresis
  - colorimetric
  - iso-electric focussing
- A labile glycosylated haemoglobin (pre-$A_{1c}$)
  - forms with acute rise in blood glucose
  - co-elutes with $HbA_{1c}$ down column
  - can add 1–3% to glycosylated haemoglobin fractions
  - can be removed by prior incubation of red cells or dialysis
- False-high values of glycosylated haemoglobins — with column methods
  - presence of HbF:  pregnancy
                      thalassaemia
                      HbH
  - carbamylated haemoglobin (uraemia)
- False-low values
  - haemolytic anaemia
  - HbS
  - HbC

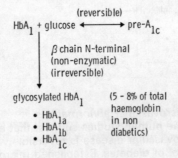

$$HbA_1 + glucose \xleftrightarrow{\text{(reversible)}} pre\text{-}A_{1c}$$

β chain N-terminal
(non-enzymatic)
(irreversible)

glycosylated $HbA_1$        (5 - 8% of total
                            haemoglobin
- $HbA_{1a}$                in non
- $HbA_{1b}$                diabetics)
- $HbA_{1c}$

**Fig. 5.4**

## MACROANGIOPATHY

Diabetes magnifies the risk factors associated with atheromatous disease. Contributory factors may be similar to those for microangiopathy
- hyperlipidaemia with decreased HDL (protective)
- increased blood viscosity and hypercoaguability
- hypertension
- prostaglandin/thromboxane imbalance
- ? altered endothelial cell metabolism

Results in
- coronary arterial disease
- peripheral vascular disease

Diabetic cardiomyopathy results from
- coronary atheromatous disease
- microangiopathy
- perivascular and interstitial fibrosis
- abnormal cardiac metabolism

Causes of death in diabetes <50 years of age
- myocardial infarction                        30%
- cerebrovascular and other arterial           10%
- renal disease                                20%
- ketoacidosis                                 15%
- hypoglycaemia                                 5%
- other non-diabetic causes                    20%

## DIABETIC NEUROPATHY

Absence of uniform criteria for diagnosis of neuropathy makes studies on incidence difficult.
- 90% of diabetes with duration of disease >10 years have some evidence of neuropathy.
- Severity of neuropathy can be independent of other diabetic complications.
- Segmental demyelination is chief histological feature.

*Aetiology — probably multifactorial*
- ? glycosylation of nerve membranes and contractile proteins in axon may impair axonal transport mechanism
- ? increased glucose metabolism to sorbitol and fructose via polyol pathway in nerve:

$$glucose \xrightarrow{\text{aldose reductase}} Sorbitol \longrightarrow Fructose$$

- sorbitol accumulation may inhibit myo-inositol synthesis, a polyhydric alcohol associated with myelination
- aldose reductase inhibitors (e.g. sorbinil) prevent sorbitol accumulation and myo-inositol deficiency and can improve some features of neuropathy
- micro- and macrovessel damage of vasa nervorum may be cause of mononeuropathies

*Polyneuropathy (mostly sensory)*
- hyperparaesthesia/paraesthesia
- absent tendon reflexes, vibration and pain sensation
- Charcot joint
- neuropathic ulcer — at pressure points

*Mononeuropathy (usually motor)*
- single nerve involvement with muscle pain and atrophy
- cranials III, VI, and VII
- ulnar, femoral, peroneal
- can resolve spontaneously

*Autonomic neuropathy*
- can be detected in 20–40% of diabetics
Cardiovascular
1. parasympathetic loss (early)
   - tachycardia
   - no bradycardia or BP elevation after Valsalva
   - no beat to beat variation on ECG during deep breathing or after standing
2. sympathetic loss (late)
   - no BP rise during handgrip
   - postural hypotension — aggravation by insulin
   - peripheral arteriovenous shunts — tissue ischaemia and oedema especially in feet
   - ? medial calcification of peripheral arteries
Gastrointestinal
- gastric stasis/vomiting
- diarrhoea — often nocturnal, rarely malabsorption (? stasis causing abnormal gut flora)
Urino-genital
- urinary retention
- impotence, retrograde ejaculation
Others
- gustatory sweating
- loss of warning symptoms of hypoglycaemia
- anaesthetic deaths

**Treatment**
Painful neuropathy
- analgesics
- carbamazepine, phenytoin may be helpful
- continuous subcutaneous insulin infusion
- aldose reductase inhibitors are being evaluated

Postural hypotension symptoms
- fludrocortisone 0.1–0.3 mg daily
- indomethacin, β-blocker pindolol have been used with varying success
- postural symptoms may abate with onset of renal failure but return with dialysis or successful renal transplant
- if insulin aggravates hypotension, change timing of injections

Gastrointestinal symptoms
- metoclopramide 10 mg t.d.s. for stasis, vomiting and diarrhoea
- tetracyclines or other broad spectrum antibiotics may help diarrhoea by eradicating abnormal gut flora
- anti-diarrhoeal e.g. codeine, anti-cholinergics etc.

Bladder symptoms
- encourage frequent voiding with suprapubic pressure if required
- treat urinary infections promptly
- bladder neck resection may relieve residual urine collections

Impotence
- sexual counselling most useful as there is no cure
- penile prostheses have variable success

Gustatory sweating
- anticholinergics before meals e.g. poldine

Diabetic foot
- treat oedema with diuretics or pressure stockings; ephedrine may help some
- footwear should ensure even distribution of pressure — calluses, deformed nails removed by chiropodist
- ulceration, local infections should be treated promptly
- surgery is indicated for:
  - debridement of infected site
  - amputation of gangrenous tissue


## EYE COMPLICATIONS OF DIABETES

Conjunctiva
- non-specific and insignificant changes e.g. microaneurysms

Iris
- rubeosis iridis (new vessels on iris)
  - obstruction of aqueous drainage — glaucoma
  - bleed during cataract surgery
  - associated with proliferative retinopathy
- Argyll-Robertson pupil

Anterior chamber (aqueous humor)
- glaucoma
  - due to rubeosis irides
  - thrombotic

Lens
- dehydration, osmotic (hyperglycaemic) change
  - reversible 'opacities' due to wrinkling of lens capsule
  - myopia — hypermetropia with blood sugar control
- cataracts
  - central subcapsular
  - diffuse, nuclear
  - linear peripheral and radial
  - acute, progressive in young diabetics — usually central and bilateral

Vitreous
- haemorrhage
- retinitis proliferans
- vitreal detachment

Retina
- retinopathy
- lipaemia retinalis

Optic nerve
- optic atrophy (Diabetes Insipidus, Diabetes Mellitus, Optic Atrophy, Nerve Deafness — DIDMOAD syndrome)
- papilloedema — rare

**Diabetic retinopathy**
- Most insulin dependent diabetics have some retinopathy after 10 years of diabetes.
- Retinopathy may be present in 10% of non-insulin dependent diabetics at diagnosis; maculopathy is common (Fig. 5.5).
- Patients with retinopathy should be referred to a specialist unit for assessment and treatment (Table 5.4).
- Photocoagulation therapy destroys ischaemic retina and causes regression of new vessels and hard exudates.

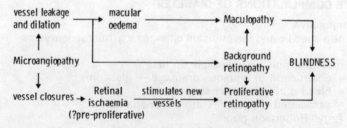

Fig. 5.5

**Table 5.4**

| Type of retinopathy | Fundoscopy | Action |
|---|---|---|
| Background | Hard exudates, microaneurysms, small haemorrhages | Check eyes 6 monthly; optimize diabetic control |
| Maculopathy | Macular oedema | Foveal vision at risk local photocoagulation |
| | Circinate exudates | if visual acuity falls |
| Pre-proliferative | Multiple 'cotton wool'spots (retinal infarcts), venular beading and loops, intra-retinal microvessel abnormality, arterial sheathing | Review frequently ? may benefit from early photocoagulation |
| Proliferative | Above + new vessels, disc new vessels | Urgent peripheral photocoagulation (medical emergency) |
| Vitreous bleeds | New vessels may be seen after clearing of haemorrhage | Peripheral photocoagulation |
| Retinitis proliferans | Fibrous new vessels attached to shrunken vitreous → retinal or macular traction | Irreversible vitrectomy may be possible in some; alert social agencies |

*Prognosis*
- Patients with visual acuity of 6/36 or worse due to diabetic retinopathy will not usually benefit from photocoagulation.
- 30% of patients with untreated disc new vessels become blind in 2 years.
- There is little evidence that hypertension, diabetic control, smoking etc. influence the course of established retinopathy.

**Diabetic nephropathy**
- diabetic nephropathy is the clinical consequence of glomerular microvessel disease in diabetics
- persistant proteinuria occurs in 10–15% of diabetics with 10 year disease duration
- 30% of IDDM develop nephropathy, though 60–90% of all diabetics have histological evidence of glomerulopathy at autopsy
- men appear to be more susceptible

*Pathology*
- all stages of progression may be present in same patient
- early glomerular:
    capillary basement membrane thickening, dilatation, closures,
    etc.; increased glomerular filtration rate (GFR) and micro-
    albuminuria are present, but reversible on achieving
    normoglycaemia
- diffuse glomerular:
    endothelial polysaccharride accumulation, basement
    membrane thickening
- nodular (Kimmelsteil-Wilson):
    specific for diabetes; homogeneously staining peripheral
    nodules that can expand to compromise glomerular capillary
    function with resultant ischaemia
- exudative:
    fibrinoid material widely present between capillary
    endothelium and basement membrane

*Clinical course* (*Fig. 5.6*)
Rate of disease progression varies widely in diabetics; when
creatinine >200 $\mu$mol/l, a linear relationship with time to 1/serum
creatinine or log serum creatinine is present in individual (Fig. 5.7)

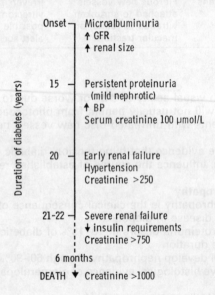

| Duration of diabetes (years) | | |
|---|---|---|
| Onset | Microalbuminuria<br>↑ GFR<br>↑ renal size | |
| 15 | Persistent proteinuria<br>(mild nephrotic)<br>↑ BP<br>Serum creatinine 100 µmol/L | |
| 20 | Early renal failure<br>Hypertension<br>Creatinine >250 | |
| 21-22 | Severe renal failure<br>↓ insulin requirements<br>Creatinine >750 | |
| 6 months | | |
| DEATH ↓ | Creatinine >1000 | |

Fig. 5.6

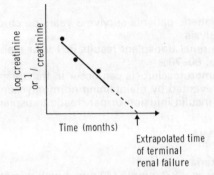

**Fig. 5.7**

*Management*
- it is essential to exclude other reversible causes of the nephrotic syndrome in young diabetics of short disease duration
- over 50% with nephropathy have proliferative retinopathy; opthalmological assessment essential
- optimal control is unlikely to reverse established pathology, but may retard progress
- urinary tract infections, hypertension should be treated promptly
- oral hypoglycaemics are probably best avoided, and insulin started
- at onset of proteinuria, 6 to 12 monthly checks on serum creatinine should be made
- Refer to local renal units *before* serum creatinine >500 $\mu$mol/l for consideration of
  1. dialysis
     - haemodialysis
     - chronic ambulatory peritoneal dialysis (now increasingly used in diabetics) — insulin can be given intraperitoneally with excellent control of diabetes
  2. renal transplantation
  3. combined renal and pancreas transplant

*Prognosis*
- 80% of those with diabetic nephropathy die with renal failure — the rest dying from ischaemic heart disease
- with renal transplantation using live donor kidney (USA figures)
  - 3 year cumulative survival in 65%, increases to 80% with HLA compatibility
  - transplant mortality increased in diabetics with ischaemic heart disease

- in Europe
  - 30% of diabetic patients survive 3 years on chronic haemodialysis
  - cadaveric renal transplant results in 1 year diabetic patient survival of 60–70%
- diabetic glomerulosclerosis can occur in transplanted kidney — it can be prevented by maintaining normoglycaemia with continuous insulin infusion or pancreatic transplant

## HYPOGLYCAEMIA

### Diagnostic criteria
- plasma glucose <2.2 mmol/l (40 mg%) with symptoms that quickly reverse after giving glucose
- fasting hypoglycaemia, or with food deprivation, suggests organic disease e.g. insulinoma
- reactive hypoglycaemia in response to meals or drugs is rarely due to organic disease

### Causes
Hyperinsulinism
- exogenous administration of insulin
- endogenous
  - pancreatic insulinoma
  - nesidioblastosis — β cell hyperplasia of infancy
  - reactive
    - dumping syndrome
    - leucine hypersensitivity
    - carbohydrate loading
    - infants of diabetic mothers
    - oral hypoglycaemics
    - early stages of diabetes
  - ? acute pancreatitis, liver and renal failure
- increased glucose consumption or loss
  - ? large neoplasms
  - excessive exercise
  - haemodialysis using glucose free solution
  - renal glycosuria
- decreased glucose production or availability
  - severe starvation
  - ketotic hypoglycaemia of infancy
  - hepatocellular disease
  - decreased gluconeogenic hormones
    - Addisons disease
    - hypopituitarism
    - hypothyroidism

- inborn errors of metabolism
  - galactosaemia (galactose-1-phosphate uridyltransferase deficiency)
  - fructose intolerance (fructose-1-phosphate aldolase deficiency)
  - glycogen storage diseases (glucose-6-phosphatase, liver phosphorylase, and debranching enzyme deficiencies)
  - deficiency of enzymes of gluconeogenesis
- ? increased somatomedin (insulin growth factors I and II)
  - neoplasia
    - mesenchymal tumours
    - hepatoma
    - adrenocortical carcinoma
    - gastrointestinal malignancies
    - myeloproliferative disorders
- ? insulin binding antibodies
- drugs
  - alcohol
  - sulphonylureas
  - salicylates
  - propranolol — also prolongs hypoglycaemia, by inhibiting the gluconeogenic effect of increased catecholamine secretion

**Symptoms**
These vary with rate and duration of blood glucose fall

| Acute (fall <1/2 h) | Subacute (fall >1 h) | Chronic (chronically low glucose) |
|---|---|---|
| hunger | sleepiness | psychosis |
| anxiety, restlessness | intoxication behaviour | dementia |
| tachycardia, palpitations | amnesia | hypoglycaemic neuropathy |
| sweatiness | semiconsciousness | |
| tremor | transient hemiplegia | |
| dysarthria | | |
| dizziness | | |
| epilepsy in children | | |

Acute symptoms are mostly due to increased sympathomimetic activity and can be masked with β-blockers, though sweating is not affected. Acute hypoglycaemia is commonly due to insulin use or is 'reactive'.

Subacute or chronic hypoglycaemia is usually due to an insulinoma.

## Investigations
- Measure glucose, insulin and C-peptide in blood sample taken at onset of symptoms which may occur spontaneously or during a prolonged 10–48 hour fast
- A low blood glucose with inappropriately elevated insulin and C-peptide suggests endogenous hyperinsulinism usually due to an insulinoma. Pro-insulin levels are elevated with insulinomas
- Elevated insulin with low C-peptide levels suggests exogenous (factitious) insulin administration
- Stimulation tests e.g. fish insulin, tolbutamide, oral glucose are usually unnecessary as 90% of insulinomas are revealed during prolonged fasting
- Exclude other causes:
  - check endocrine function
  - liver function
  - ultrasound or computerized tomography for mesenchymal tumours

## Treatment
- Acute symptoms should be reversed with intravenous glucose
- If possible treat underlying cause
- insulinomas should be excised, or cytotoxics such as streptozotocin used
- Diazoxide 200–600 mg/day inhibits insulin release but causes salt and water retention, which is reduced by chlorthiazide. Diazoxide can be used as a palliative for insulinomas
- Reactive hypoglycaemia may respond to small and frequent carbohydrate meals

## LACTIC ACIDOSIS

### Diagnostic criteria
Metabolic acidosis with arterial blood pH < 7.25 and serum lactate >5 mmol/l (normal 0.4–1.3) or suspect if anion gap (plasma $[Na^+ + K^+] - [HCO_3^- + Cl^-]$) > 18 mmol/l (normal 10–18).

*Other causes of anion gap*
- diabetic ketoacidosis
- uraemia
- hyperchloraemic acidosis
- salicylate overdose
- drug-induced acidosis

**Pathophysiology**

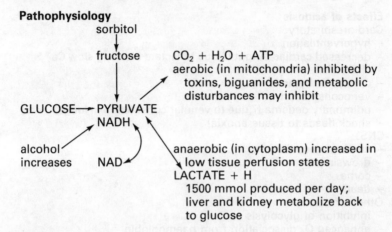

**Causes**

Type A (decreased tissue perfusion) — commonest type of lactic acidosis
- hypotensive or 'shock' states
- arterial hypoxia
- tissue anoxia

Type B (no initial circulation impairment or tissue anoxia; arterial $pO_2$ is normal)
- diseases
  - diabetic ketoacidosis
  - liver and kidney failure
  - infection
  - leukaemia, reticuloses
  - pancreatitis
- drugs
  - biguanides (less with metformin) in presence of renal dysfunction
  - energy substrates: alcohol, sorbitol, fructose
  - poisoning: methanol, salicylates, early in paracetamol poisoning
- hereditary disease
  - liver fructose 1,6 diphosphatase deficiency
  - glycogen storage type I
  - methylmalonic aciduria
  - Leigh's encephalomyopathy

**Effects of acidosis**

Cardiorespiratory:
- hyperventilation
- decreased cardiac output (? due to lactate blocking slow $Ca^{++}$ channels)
- cardiac arrhythmia
- venoconstriction
- pulmonary oedema (? due to venular constriction in lungs)
- shock (leads to tissue anoxia)

CNS:
- cerebral vasodilation
- drowsiness
- coma
- death

Other effects:
- inhibition of glycolysis
- enhanced $O_2$ dissociation from haemoglobin
- reduced hepatic clearance of lactate

**Treatment**
- Type A
  - treat precipitating events
  - correct hypovolaemia, hypoxia, hypertension etc.
- Type B
  - haemodialysis, peritoneal dialysis avoids the hazards associated with $NaHCO_3$
  - insulin-glucose infusion — ?useful for biguanide poisoning
  - $NaHCO_3$ 10 mmol/hour intravenously to maintain pH 7.35–7.42 but complications of this therapy include:
    - Na and fluid overload may cause pulmonary oedema
    - tetany
    - hypokalaemia
    - impaired $O_2$ dissociation from haemoglobin — increased tissue anoxia
    - cerebrospinal pH in brain may fall leading to coma
    - alkalosis 'overshoot'

*Other forms of therapy*
- sodium dichloroacetate — activates pyruvate dehydrogenase which lowers lactic acid production
- prostacyclin — dilates pre-capillary sphincters to improve local tissue perfusion

**Prognosis**
- Type A is commoner form and has worst prognosis because of precipitating factors
- lactate >9 mmol/l is associated with 75 to 100% mortality
- phenformin acidosis — 50% mortality — but now rare as drug is used less
- paracetamol overdose and other poisons are now commoner causes of Type B

# 6. Gastrointestinal regulatory peptides

## PHYSIOLOGY

**Gastrin**
Localisation:
- G-cells of antrum
Function:
- circulating hormone
Release:
- food in stomach, ? bombesin
- inhibited by low pH
- vagus
Actions:
- stimulates acid and pepsin secretion
- stimulates gastric mucosal blood flow
- trophic effect on stomach, small intestine and pancreas
Clinical significance:
- raised levels with atrophic gastritis (especially pernicious anaemia)
- raised levels with any other cause of acid hyposecretion
- raised levels with gastrinoma (Zollinger-Ellison syndrome)

**Secretin**
Localisation:
- S cells of duodenal and jejunal mucosa
Function:
- circulating hormone
Release:
- duodenal acidification
Actions:
- stimulates water and bicarbonate secretion from exocrine pancreas
- stimulates hepatic bile and intestinal secretion
- inhibits gastric acid secretion (? via SRIF release)
Clinical significance:
- impaired release in coeliac disease, ? in duodenitis
- elevated in acid hypersecretion e.g. Zollinger-Ellison syndrome

## Cholecystokinin (CCK)

Localisation:
- I cells of duodenal and jejunal mucosa
- cerebral tissue

Function:
- circulating hormone
- neurotransmitter in CNS and other tissues

Release:
- protein and fat in duodenum

Actions:
- stimulates pancreatic enzyme secretion and gall bladder contraction
- stimulates relaxation of sphincter of Oddi and intestinal motor activity

Clinical significance:
- used in cholecystography and assessment of pancreatic exocrine function (analogues)
- ? raised levels in steatorrhoea

## Pancreatic polypeptide (PP)

Localisation:
- pancreas

Function:
- circulating hormone

Release:
- CCK, secretin, neurotensin, bombesin
- cholinergic stimulation e.g. hypoglycaemia

Actions:
- inhibits pancreatic exocrine secretion and bile output
- inhibits motilin secretion

Clinical significance
- raised levels in diabetes mellitus, certain pancreatic endocrine tumours
- low levels in pancreatic exocrine deficiency

## Gastric inhibitory peptide (GIP)

Localisation:
- K cells in small intestine, especially duodenum and jejunum

Function:
- circulating hormone:

Release:
- absorbed nutrients, especially fat and glucose

Actions:
- inhibits gastric acid secretion
- stimulates small intestine secretion, mesenteric blood flow, lipoprotein lipase activity
- potentiates insulin release

Clinical significance:
- ? involved in enteroinsular axis

**Motilin**
Localisation:
- mucosal endocrine cells in small intestine, especially proximal jejunum

Function:
- circulating hormone

Release:
- high fat meal
- gastric distension
- cholinergic nerves
- inhibited by protein and carbohydrate meal
- inhibited by PP

Actions:
- stimulates gastric and intestinal contractions
- controls gastric emptying and colonic motility

Clinical significance:
- raised levels in diarrhoea from any cause

**Neurotensin (NT)**
Localisation:
- N cells in small intestine, especially ileal mucosa
- CNS, especially hypothalamus and basal ganglia

Function:
- circulating hormone
- neurotransmitter

Release:
- ingestion of food, especially fat

Actions:
- inhibits gastric motility and secretion
- stimulates pancreatic water and bicarbonate secretion
- stimulates PP

Clinical significance:
- increased release in dumping syndrome and ileojejunal bypass
- raised levels in some pancreatic endocrine tumours, especially vipoma

**Enteroglucagon**
Localisation:
- EG cells in intestinal mucosa, especially ileum and colon

Function:
- circulating hormone

Release:
- ingestion of fat or carbohydrate

Actions:
- ? general trophic effect on gastrointestinal tract

Clinical significance:
- raised levels in coeliac disease, cystic fibrosis, tropical sprue
- high levels with enteroglucagonoma

## Somatostatin (SRIF)
Localisation:
- δ cells in pancreas and antrum
- CNS, especially hypothalamus

Function:
- paracrine hormone
- neurotransmitter
- ? circulating hormone

Release:
- several gastrointestinal hormones

Actions:
- inhibits gut and pancreatic hormone secretion
- inhibits alimentary exocrine secretion
- inhibits growth hormone and TSH release

Clinical significance:
- modulates gut hormone secretory response to other stimuli
- raised levels in somatostatinoma and certain other pancreatic endocrine tumours
- possible uses in management of peptic ulcer haemorrhage and diabetes mellitus (under investigation)

## Bombesin (GRP in mammals)
Localisation:
- nerve fibres in stomach and upper small intestine
- CNS, lung

Function:
- neurotransmitter

Actions:
- stimulates gut and pancreatic hormone secretion
- stimulates alimentary exocrine secretion
- stimulates smooth muscle contractility e.g. gall bladder

Clinical significance:
- stimulator of gut hormone secretion
- high circulating levels in some oat-cell carcinomas, medullary thyroid carcinomas

## Vasoactive intestinal peptide (VIP)
Localisation:
- neural elements throughout entire gastrointestinal tract
- CNS, urogenital tract, lung

Function:
- neurotransmitter

Actions
- stimulates small intestine secretion, pancreatic bicarbonate secretion, insulin secretion, hepatic glycogenolysis
- inhibits gastric acid secretion
- causes vasodilatation, smooth muscle relaxation

Clinical significance:
- high circulating levels in vipomas (Werner-Morrison syndrome)
- increased VIPergic nerves in Crohn's disease
- decreased VIPergic nerves in Hirschsprung's disease, Chagas' disease

**Substance P**
Localisation:
- neural elements throughout entire gastrointestinal tract
- autonomic nerves in pancreas, eye, urogenital tract
- CNS
Function:
- neurotransmitter
Actions:
- stimulates pancreatic exocrine secretion, salivary gland secretion, small intestine water absorption
- stimulates pancreatic glucagon release
- inhibits insulin release, hepatic bile
- causes smooth muscle contraction, diarrhoea, bronchoconstriction, hypotension, flushing
Clinical significance:
- involved in pain perception
- high circulating levels with some carcinoid tumours
- decreased substance P-containing nerves in Hirschsprung's disease, Chagas' disease

**Enkephalin**
Location:
- nerve fibres in antrum, duodenum and pancreas
- CNS
Functions:
- neurotransmitter
Actions:
- inhibits gastric emptying and intestinal motility
- inhibits pancreatic secretion
- ? augments gastric secretion
Clinical significance:
- unknown

**Thyrotrophin-releasing hormone (TRH)**
Location:
- nerve fibres in antrum, duodenum and pancreas
- hypothalamus
Function:
- neurotransmitter

Actions:
- inhibits gastric acid secretion and intestinal motility
- inhibits glucose and xylose absorption
- stimulates TSH release

Clinical significance:
- unknown

## Peptide YY (PYY)

Location:
- mucosal endocrine cells in intestine, mainly colon

Function:
- circulating hormone

Release:
- not reported

Actions:
- inhibits gastric acid secretion
- hypertensive

Clinical significance:
- unknown

## Peptide HI (PHI)

Location:
- nerve fibres in GI tract, CNS, urogenital tract, lung, etc.

Function:
- ? neurotransmitter
- probably co-secreted with VIP

Actions:
- stimulates small intestinal secretion
- exhibits other VIP-like actions

Clinical significance:
- elevated levels in Werner-Morrison syndrome

## Neuropeptide Y (NPY)

Location:
- nerve fibres in CNS, heart, urogenital tract

Function:
- neurotransmitter

Actions:
- hypertensive
- stimulates smooth muscle contractility
- inhibits pancreatic exocrine secretion

Clinical significance:
- elevated levels in phaeochromocytoma

## Control of gastric acid secretion

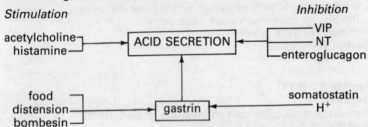

## Control of pancreatic exocrine secretion

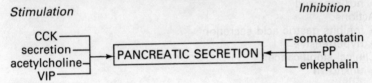

## CLINICAL DISORDERS

### Zollinger-Ellison syndrome

*Definition*
- peptic ulcer disease, gastric acid hypersecretion and non-β-islet cell tumour (usually)

*Pathophysiology*

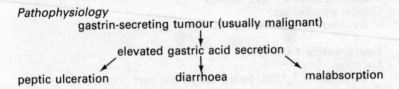

*Clinical features*
- recurrent severe peptic ulceration
- multiple peptic ulcers
- ectopic locations of peptic ulcers
- diarrhoea
- multiple endocrine neoplasia type I

*Diagnosis*
- hypergastrinaemia
- gastric acid hypersecretion
- demonstration of islet cell tumour or hyperplasia (pancreas or duodenum; ± metastases)

*Differential diagnosis of hypergastrinaemia*
- Zollinger-Ellison syndrome
- pernicious anaemia
- chronic atrophic gastritis
- chronic renal failure
- gastric carcinoma
- phaeochromocytoma
- rheumatoid arthritis
- vitiligo

*Management*
- surgical
  - ablation of acid-secreting tissue + removal of tumour
  - hepatic artery embolization
- medical
  - $H_2$ receptor antagonists
  - ATPase inhibitors
  - streptozotocin

**Werner-Morrison syndrome**

*Definition*
- watery diarrhoea, hypokalaemia, hypochlorhydria, pancreatic islet cell tumours (80%) or sympathetic chain (20%)

*Pathophysiology*

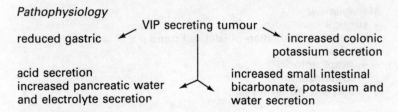

reduced gastric

VIP secreting tumour

increased colonic potassium secretion

acid secretion
increased pancreatic water
and electrolyte secretion

increased small intestinal
bicarbonate, potassium and
water secretion

*Clinical features*
- profuse watery diarrhoea
- marked hypokalaemia
- flushing (occasional)
- hypercalcaemia
- gastric acid hyposecretion

*Diagnosis*
- elevated plasma VIP (usual)
- hypokalaemia
- hyperglycaemia/hypercalcaemia
- demonstration of pancreatic islet cell tumour or hyperplasia
  (± metastases; occasionally ectopic)

*Management*
- surgical
  - removal or ablation of islet cell tumour
- medical
  - streptozotocin
  - corticosteroids

## Glucagonoma

*Definition*
- α-cell pancreatic tumour

*Clinical features*
- profound weight loss (marked catabolism)
- variable diabetes mellitus
- necrotising migratory erythema
- anaemia (normochromic, normocytic)
- stomatitis, glossitis
- pulmonary embolism (common cause of death)

*Diagnosis*
- elevated plasma glucagon
  demonstration of α-cell islet tumour or hyperplasia
  (± metastases)

*Management*
- surgical
  - removal or ablation of islet cell tumour
- medical
  - streptozotocin
  - somatostatin
  - oral zinc (for skin rash)

## Insulinoma

*Definition*
- β-cell pancreatic tumour (90% benign)

*Clinical features*
- those of hypoglycaemia (see Ch. 5)

*Diagnosis*
- inappropriately elevated insulin levels during hypoglycaemia
- demonstration of β-cell islet tumour (usually benign)

*Management*
- surgical
  - removal or ablation of islet cell tumour
- medical
  - streptozotocin
  - somatostatin
  - frequent eating

## Somatostatinoma

*Definition*
- δ cell pancreatic tumour

*Clinical features*
- very non-specific features
- diabetes mellitus
- hypochlorhydria
- gallstones
- steatorrhoea

*Diagnosis*
- elevated plasma somatostatin
- decreased plasma insulin and glucagon
- demonstration of D-cell islet tumour (± metastases)

*Management*
- surgical
  - removal or ablation of islet cell tumour
- medical
  - streptozotocin

## Carcinoid syndrome

*Definition*
- enterochromaffin tumour secreting biologically active amines

*Clinical features*
- due to secretion of biologically active amines (5-HT, bradykinin, etc.)
- flushing of skin
- diarrhoea
- cardiac lesions e.g. tricuspid valve disorder, right heart failure
- asthma
- pellagra-like skin lesions
- features due to ectopic peptide hormone production e.g. Cushing's syndrome

*Diagnosis*
- urinary 5-HIAA may be elevated
- demonstration of ectopic hormone production e.g. ACTH
- localisation of tumour
  - thymus
  - lung
  - pancreas
  - gut

*Management*
- surgical removal
- cyproheptadine, methysergide, cytotoxic chemotherapy

# 7. Adrenal disorders

## ADRENAL CORTEX

### Physiology

1. *Steroid synthesis* (Fig. 7.1)

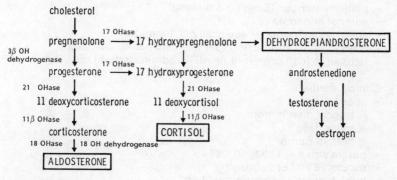

**Fig. 7.1**

2. *Control*
   cortisol
   - secretion controlled by ACTH
   - negative feedback on pituitary
   - circadian variation
   aldosterone
   - secretion controlled by renin-angiotensin system
   dehydroepiandrosterone
   - secretion controlled by ACTH
   - circadian rhythm unclear
3. *Actions*
   cortisol
   - promotes gluconeogenesis
   - decreases glucose uptake
   - inhibits lipogenesis
   - inhibits collagen formation

- impairs intestinal calcium absorption
- resorbs bone
- impairs GH release and actions
- impairs leucocyte action and immune response
- weak mineralocorticoid effect

aldosterone
- promotes renal sodium retention
- promotes renal potassium excretion

dehydroepiandrosterone
- minor contribution to androgens and oestrogens (see ch. 8)
- oestrogen contribution of most importance after menopause

## CORTISOL HYPERSECRETION (Cushing's syndrome)

*Causes*
- pituitary tumour (Cushing's disease)
- adrenal adenoma
- adrenal carcinoma — especially childhood
- ectopic ACTH production (oat cell carcinoma; carcinoid)
- iatrogenic (corticosteroid or ACTH administration)

*Clinical features*
- obesity
  - truncal distribution
  - moon face
  - buffalo hump
- purple striae — collagen loss
- excessive and easy bruising
- hypertension — sodium retention
- peripheral oedema
- proximal myopathy
- diabetes mellitus
- osteoporosis
- hirsutism
- growth retardation
- conjunctival oedema
- amenorrhoea/impotence
- susceptibility to infection
- psychiatric disturbance
- rapid onset with adrenal carcinoma/ectopic ACTH

**Investigations**

|  | Adrenal tumour | Pituitary tumour | Ectopic tumour |
|---|---|---|---|
| Sex | F > M | F > M | M > F |
| Plasma cortisol (loss of circadian rhythm) | ↑ | ↑ | ↑ ↑ |
| Plasma ACTH (loss of circadian rhythm) | ↓ | ↑ | ↑ ↑ |
| diabetic GTT | + | ± | + + |
| Dexamethasone suppression | − | + | − |
| Metyrapone test | − | + + | ± |

- plasma potassium/bicarbonate
- radiology
  - pituitary fossa ± CT scanning
  - lateral spine — osteoporosis
- adrenal imaging
  - ultrasound
  - CT scanning
  - cholesterol scanning
- ectopic tumour
  - chest radiograph ± CT scanning
  - pancreatic ultrasound ± CT scanning
- selective tumours sampling for ACTH
- general pituitary investigations (including insulin stress test)

*Differential diagnosis*
- simple obesity
- depression
- alcoholism

*Management*
- adrenal tumour
  - surgical removal
  - metyrapone, o.p'DDD
- pituitary tumour
  - (see Ch. 2)
  - ablation — surgery/irradiation
  - chemotherapy
- ectopic tumour
  - removal of tumour
  - bilateral adrenalectomy
  - metyrapone

## ALDOSTERONE HYPERSECRETION

### Causes
1. *primary*
   - adrenal adenoma (Conn's syndrome)
   - adrenal hyperplasia
   - adrenal carcinoma (very rare)
2. *secondary*
   - hypertension
     - essential
     - accelerated
   - diuretic therapy
   - nephrotic syndrome
   - cirrhosis
   - congestive cardiac failure
   - salt-losing nephropathy
   - renal tubular acidosis
   - Bartter's syndrome
   - renin hypersecretion
   - renal tumours

### Clinical features
1. *primary*
   - F > M
   - features of hypertension
   - hypokalaemia
     - polyuria
     - neuromuscular problems
     - impaired GTT
2. *secondary*
   - features of underlying cause ± hypertension, hypokalaemia

### Investigations
- plasma/urine electrolytes
- plasma aldosterone elevation
- plasma renin
- suppressed in primary
- elevated in secondary
- adrenal imaging

### Differential diagnosis
- Cushing's syndrome
- Congenital adrenal hyperplasia (see Ch. 8)
- some cases of hypertension
- drugs e.g. liquorice, carbenoxolone

**Management**
1. *primary*
   - removal of tumour
   - spironolactone
2. *secondary*
   - treatment of underlying cause

## ADRENOGENITAL SYNDROMES (see Ch. 8)

## ADRENAL HYPOSECRETION
1. *Cortisol hyposecretion*
   - Addison's disease
   - adrenalectomy
   - pituitary failure
   - adrenogenital syndromes
2. *Aldosterone hyposecretion*
   - Addison's disease
   - adrenalectomy
   - impaired renin-angiotensin system
   - inborn error

**Addison's disease**
*Causes*
- autoimmune disease
- tuberculosis
- amyloidosis
- haemochromatosis
- fungal infections
- haemorrhage
- vascular disruption
*Clinical features*
- skin pigmentation
- hypotension
- weakness
- anorexia and weight loss
- nausea and vomiting
- amenorrhoea, loss of body hair in women
- vitiligo
*Investigations*
- hyponatraemia/hyperkalaemia
- hypoglycaemia
- plasma cortisol low
- plasma ACTH elevated (unless pituitary failure)
- synacthen test impaired
- anaemia, eosinophilia

*Management*
acute
- intravenous corticosteroids
- intravenous fluid volume replacement
chronic
- oral cortisol replacement
- oral mineralocorticoid replacement
- medical warning card, bracelet etc.
- increased cortisol requirement with surgery, infection etc.

## ADRENAL MEDULLA

### Physiology
1. *Synthesis* (Fig. 7.2)

Synthesis

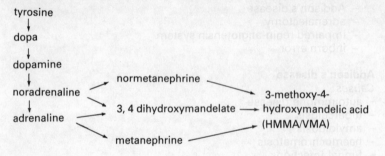

**Fig. 7.2**

2. *Control*
    - sympathetic innervation — controlled by hypothalamus and brain stem
    - hypoglycaemia stimulates release
    - pharmacological agonists and blocking agents
3. *Actions*
    - via cyclic AMP
    - stimulation of adrenergic receptors
    - cardiovascular effects — increased heart rate, BP, skeletal blood flow + peripheral vasoconstriction
    - lipolysis and FFA liberation
    - glycogenolysis — increased blood glucose
    - skeletal muscle — affects slow-contracting muscle
    - gastrointestinal tract — relaxes smooth muscle

**Phaeochromocytoma**

*Definition*
Tumour arising from chromaffin cells producing excess catecholamines. May be benign or malignant.

*Causes*
- adrenal phaeochromocytoma
- ganglioneuroma
- multiple endocrine neoplasia types II and III

*Clinical features*
- paroxysmal hypertension
- hypertension with paroxysmal attacks of headache, sweating, pallor, palpitations
- diabetes mellitus
- neurofibromas, neuromas
- vitiligo, cafe-au-lait spots
- family history
- other components of multiple endocrine neoplasia

*Investigations*
- Increased 24 hour urinary metabolites — VMA, metanephrine, normetanephrine, dopamine (if malignant)
- plasma adrenaline, noradrenaline raised
- tumour localization — selective venous sampling, arteriography, CT scanning, [131I]-m-iodobenzylguanidine scanning
- plasma calcium — if raised, check PTH level
- plasma calcitonin

*Management*
acute
- α-blockers, ± β-blockers later
chronic
- surgical removal
- α and β blockade
- alphamethyltyrosine

# 8. Disorders of sexual development and reproduction

## ABNORMALITIES OF OVARIAN FUNCTION

### Physiology
Ovum production and female sex steroid synthesis are linked to the menstrual cycle (Figs. 8.1, 8.2)

At birth — 2 million oocytes
Puberty — 1/2 million oocytes
Postmenopause — no oocytes

Genetically determined spontaneous atresia accounts for most of the loss of the oocytes. 15–20 are lost in early follicular phase

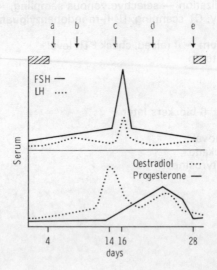

Fig. 8.1

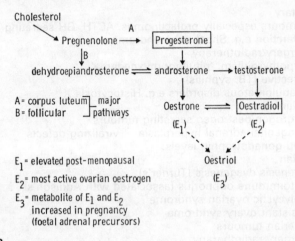

Cholesterol

A = corpus luteum ⎤ major
B = follicular ⎦ pathways

$E_1$ = elevated post-menopausal
$E_2$ = most active ovarian oestrogen
$E_3$ = metabolite of $E_1$ and $E_2$
      increased in pregnancy
      (foetal adrenal precursors)

**Fig. 8.2**

1. Under influence of FSH, several potential follicles develop, but the most efficient producer of oestrogen increases its FSH receptors, favouring its own survival while others atrese. FSH stimulates LH receptor formation.
2. FSH rise is inhibited by oestradiol. LH is inhibited at low serum oestradiol levels, but is stimulated at higher serum oestradiol levels.
3. LH surge occurs when serum oestradiol >750pmol/l for 2 days; follicular wall ruptures and ova extruded (prostaglandins may be involved). Corpus luteum forms and ova traverses fallopian tubes.
4. LH stimulates corpus luteum to increase progesterone to >25nmol/l if ovulation has occurred. Progesterone inhibits LH and FSH.
5. Absence of conception results in atresia of the corpus luteum with decreased steroid output. Menstruation with endometrial shedding.

### Female hypogonadism

*Causes*
Low gonadotrophin levels:
- hypothalamic
  - psychological stress, starvation e.g. anorexia nervosa
  - systemic illness
  - GnRH deficiency (Kallman's syndrome)
  - hypothalamic tumours e.g. craniopharyngioma
  - radiotherapy

- pituitary
    - tumours especially prolactinomas, ACTH, GH secreting
    - infarction e.g. Sheehan's syndrome
    - surgery/radiotherapy
    - hypothyroidism, 'pituitary myxoedema'
    - infective (TB, syphilis)
    - granulomatous disorders e.g. Histocytosis X
- ovarian/adrenal
    - androgen/oestrogen secreting tumours
    - congenital adrenal hyperplasia — viralizing defects
Elevated gonadotrophin levels:
- ovarian
    - agenesis/dysgenesis (Turner's)
    - autoimmune oophoritis (associated with Addison's)
    - polycystic ovarian syndrome
    - resistant ovary syndrome
    - ovarian tumours
    - surgery/radiotherapy
    - congenital adrenal hyperplasia e.g. 17-hydroxylase defect
Miscellaneous:
- interesex/chromosomal defects
- uterine/vaginal abnormalities may interfere with menses

*Clinical presentations*
- failure to attain puberty
- varying pubertal changes but absent menarche (primary amenorrhoea)
- absence of menses (for six months or 3 cycles) in previously menstruating woman (secondary amenorrhoea)
- infertility, menopausal symptoms etc.

**Hirsutism**

*Definitions*
Hirsutism:  Excess body or facial hair in female — wide subjective variation
Virilization: Clitoromegaly, male-pattern baldness, increased muscle bulk, breast atrophy, deepening of voice and hirsutes in female

*Aetiology*
Hirsutism and virilization reflect increased androgen effect in female

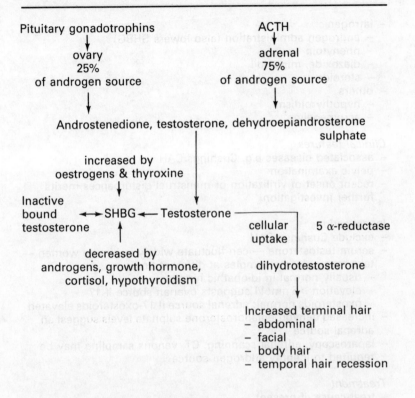

Pituitary gonadotrophins
↓
ovary
25%
of androgen source

ACTH
↓
adrenal
75%
of androgen source

↓

Androstenedione, testosterone, dehydroepiandrosterone
sulphate

increased by
oestrogens & thyroxine
↓

Inactive
bound ← → SHBG ← Testosterone
testosterone ↑

decreased by
androgens, growth hormone,
cortisol, hypothyroidism

cellular    5 α-reductase
uptake

dihydrotestosterone

Increased terminal hair
- abdominal
- facial
- body hair
- temporal hair recession

SHBG: sex hormone binding globulin
 - liver synthesis
 - 3× greater binding for testosterone than oestrogen
 - binds >99% circulatory testosterone

*Causes of hirsutism*
- idiopathic (90%)
 - ? constitutionally increased androgen secretion and/or
   increased peripheral sensitivity i.e. racial, genetic factors
- ovarian
 - polycystic ovarian syndrome
 - tumours (androgen) — arrhenoblastoma, luteoma
- adrenal
 - Cushings syndrome
 - adrenal tumours — usually malignant
 - mild congenital adrenal hyperplasia (CAH)

- iatrogenic
  - androgen administration (also lowers SHBG)
  - phenytoin
  - diazoxide, minoxidil
  - steroids
- others
  - hypothyroidism
  - acromegaly

*Clinical features*
- associated diseases e.g. Cushings/CAH
- pelvic examination
- recent onset of virilization or menstrual disturbances merits further investigation

*Investigations*
- exclude Cushings/CAH
- serum testosterone — can fluctuate widely in hirsute women — take many plasma samples at different times
  - usually normal in idiopathic hirsute
  - elevation >5 nmol/l suggests ovarian source if 17-oxosteroids normal; adrenal source if 17-oxosteroids elevated
- increased dehydroepiandrosterone sulphate levels suggest an adrenal source
- laparoscopy, adrenal scanning, CT, venous sampling may be required to identify androgen source

*Treatment*
- treat cause, if present
- adrenal and ovarian sources of androgens are suppressed with prednisolone and oestrogens which will also increase testosterone binding to SHBG
- anti-androgen and anti-gonadotrophin cyproterone acetate can be used but may induce feminization of male fetus therefore oral contraception regimen essential i.e. cyproterone acetate 100–200 mg from 5th to 14th day of menstrual cycle with oestrogen given from 5th to 25th day of cycle. This treatment is not without hazard and therefore should be supervised
- cosmetic measures are the safest
  - bleaching, shaving, depilatory creams, or electrolysis

*Prognosis*
- stopping treatment will result in recurrence of hirsutes

### Polycystic ovarian syndrome

Heterogenous disorder of steroidal-hypothalamic-pituitary feedback resulting in chronic anovulation.

Commonest cause of hirsutes with menstrual dysfunction. Aetiology of primary disorder unknown; can be inherited X-linked dominant (Fig. 8.3).

- increased androgen secretion from ovary and possibly adrenal gland is present
- chronic oestrogen elevation (mainly oestrone) stimulates pituitary LH release (positive feedback) but suppresses FSH to levels which induce only partial follicular growth. Androgens also inhibit follicular maturation
- hyperthecosis (stromal hyperplasia) is the result of anovulation

*Investigations*
- serum LH, FSH, androgens
- laparoscopy if necessary

Polycystic ovarian syndrome can be secondary to:
- Cushings disease
- congenital adrenal hyperplasia
- ovarian hyperthecosis
- androgen secreting tumour
- hyper/hypothyroidism
- hyperprolactinaemia + LH hypersecretion

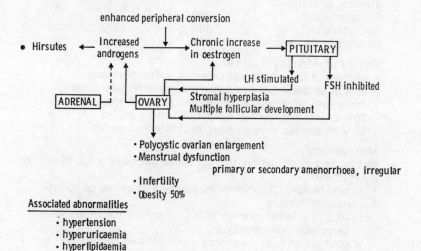

**Fig. 8.3**

*Treatment*
- medical:
  - clomiphene (anti-oestrogen) increases FSH and aids ovulation
  - pergonal (human menopausal gonadotrophin) can be used, but human pituitary FSH preferred
- surgical:
  - ovarian wedge resection can be curative; mechanism:
    ? reduction in local androgens
    ? reduction in ovarian 'inhibin' permitting FSH to increase
    ? increased intra-ovarian blood flow and exposure of gonadal tissue to gonadotrophins

*Prognosis*
- appropriate treatment with restoration of menses and fertility occurs in 60–80%

## Disorders of fertility

*Infertility*
Absence of conception after 1 year of unprotected sexual intercourse in a couple desiring pregnancy.
   Primary infertility: no previous conception.
   Secondary infertility: history of previously documented conception.

*Incidence*
10–20% of couples
Female causes:          40%
Male causes:            40%
Indeterminate causes:   20%

Causes of infertility (Fig. 8.4)
- azoospermia commonest cause of infertility in men
- 40% of all causes due to pelvic disease in female, most commonly tubal abnormalities and endometriosis
- 15% of infertile women have anovulatory cycles
- 50% of infertile women have hyperprolactinaemia

*Management*
History and examination, though cause not usually found at initial assessment
1. sexual history: technique, frequency and timing of coitus
2. menstrual history
   - 40% of infertile women with primary amenorrhoea have karyotype abnormalities
   - post-pill or post pregnancy amenorrhoea should alert to hyperprolactinaemia
3. clinical evidence of hypogonadism, endocrine disorders, systemic disease
4. pelvic examination in women, and genital examinations in men are mandatory

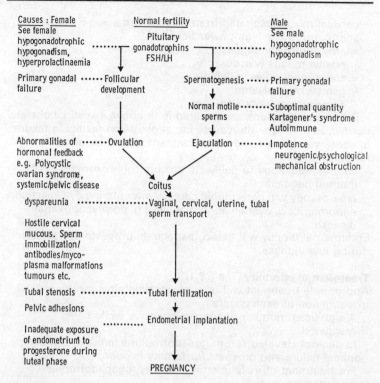

**Fig. 8.4**

*Investigations*
Order and type of investigations may be guided by history and examination but in the common situation of normal (menstruating) female and male, the following may be useful:
Sperm count
- <20 million/ml indicates suboptimal fertility, though fertility can occur at 5–10 million/ml
- immotility suggests
  - sperm antibodies in male
  - Kartageners syndrome
- azoospermia — investigate as for male hypogonadism
Ovulatory cycle indicated by
- 0.5 °C rise in basal body temperature midcycle
- serum progesterone >25 nmol/l in midluteal phase (20–24) days
Post-coital test
- examination should occur 2 days before anticipated ovulation, 2–16 hours after coitus.

- cervical mucus aspirated from cervical canal − >5 motile spermatozoa per high power field
- sperm immotility suggests:
  - hostile mucus (viscous)
  - sperm antibodies — female
  - genital mycoplasma
  - Kartageners syndrome

Pelvic investigations are required if all above investigations are normal, and 'timed' intercourse i.e. at ovulation results in failure to conceive after six cycles. Assessment should be done during follicular phase.

- contrast radiology to delineate anatomical abnormalities of internal genitalia
- laparoscopy will detect tubal patency after uterine dye injection, endometriosis, ovarian abnormalities e.g. polycystic ovarian disease

Endometrial biopsy will detect inadequate progesterone effects during luteal phase.

**Treatment of infertility** (Table 8.1)
Appropriate treatment will only be possible after careful investigation of each couple.

A significant number of couples conceive while being investigated.

In general elevated serum gonadotrophins indicate primary gonadal failure and prospect for fertility is poor.

For treatment of male infertility, see hypogonadotrophic hypogonadism (p. 139).

After exclusion of anti-sperm antibodies and genital mycoplasma infection, a hard core of 10–20% will be left in whom no cause for infertility can be found and alternatives such as adoption offered. In vitro fertilization is at present a limited and controversial procedure

**Oral contraception**
Combined preparations have one of two oestrogens and one of several progestins:

Oestrogen:                +   Progesterone:         = Combined oral contraceptive

Ethinyl oestradiol                    19 norethisterone derivatives
Mestranol (hepatic                   norethisterone
metabolism to                        norethisterone acetate
ethinyl oestradiol)                  norgestrel
                                     ethynodiol diacetate
                                     lynoestrenol
                                     (variable androgenic and oestrogenic effects occur)

**Table 8.1**

| Treatment | Indications | Method | Conception rate (%) |
|---|---|---|---|
| Clomiphene Tamoxifen ? GnRH (pulsatile) | 1. Intact hypothalamo-pituitary axis 2. Anovulatory cycle 3. Irregular menses 4. Inadequate luteal phase | 50–200 mg/day for first 5 days of cycle. Check for ovulation. HCG given mid-cycle may aid ovulation (5000 iu). | >90 |
| HMG HCG | 1. Failure of clomiphene 2. Hypothalamo-pituitary dysfunction 3. Anovulatory cycles 4. Inadequate luteal phase | HMG i.m. given until urinary oestrogen 300–400 nmol/24 h and then HCG given. | >90 |
| Bromocriptine | Hyperprolactinaemia | Increase doses to 2.5 mg t.d.s. | >90 |
| Progesterone | Inadequate luteal phase | Give daily after onset of ovulation | >30 |
| Oestrogen | Abnormal cervical mucus | 0.1 mg diethylstilboestrol on days 5–15 of cycle. | 30 |
| Cervical cup insemination | 1. Low sperm counts <20 million 2. Decreased sperm motility | Artificial insemination | 30–50 |
| Surgery | 1. Tubal disease 2. Endometriosis 3. Cervical-uterine abnormalities 4. Varicocoelectomy in men | | <50 |

*Mechanisms of contraceptive effect*
1. Oestrogen, and to a lesser extent, progesterone suppress ovulation by inhibiting GnRH release, and possibly by an indirect inhibitory effect on pituitary gonadotrophin release.
2. Progesterones alter cervical mucous composition, retarding sperm penetration.
3. Reduction of endometrial glycogen is detrimental to implantation of blastocyst.

*Metabolic effects of combined preparations*
Table 8.2 summarizes the metabolic effects and their possible
clinical consequences. In general oestrogens are implicated in
venous and carcinomatous complications, whereas
progesterones may cause arterial complications. However,
synergistic mechanisms cannot be excluded.
Risks are greatest with:
– women >35 years of age
– >50 $\mu$g oestrogen pill
– presence of risk factors
Absolute contraindications:
– thrombo-embolic tendency
– arterial disease (cerebral, cardiac, pulmonary)
– endometrial/breast carcinoma
– hepatic dysfunction
– smoking
Relative contraindications:
– hypertension
– impaired GTT
– diabetes
– prolactinomas
– migraine/epilepsy etc.
– gall stones
– hyperlipidaemias
    Though most of the metabolic effects revert to normal within a
few months of stopping, the overall risks of developing
complications may remain 4× that of women who have never
used oral contraception.

*Indications for combined oral contraception*
1. Contraception: 100% effective if used properly, and safe if
   women with risk factors excluded
2. Establishment of regular menstrual cycles (though all women
   with menstrual dysfunction need careful assessment prior to
   commencing therapy)
3. In some intersex states where a female phenotype is desired

*Follow up*
1. Routine follow up will be necessary at 3 month intervals
   during period of adjustment, or for changes in oral
   contraception, until suitable preparation found
2. Annual checks on BP, breast examination, cervical smear are
   advised for all women on oral contraception
3. Pregnancy due to inadequate compliance should be diagnosed
   early as the 'androgen' effects of the progesterone component
   may result in virilization of a female fetus
4. Drug interactions should always be considered e.g. rifampicin
   accelerates oestrogen metabolism and may result in
   pregnancy

**Table 8.2** Metabolic effects and risks of 'combined' oral contraception

| Metabolic effects | Progesterone | Oestrogen | Possible consequences |
|---|---|---|---|
| Insulin resistance | ? Major causative component | Synergistic with progesterone | Impaired GTT/Diabetes mellitus<br>? Ischaemic heart disease |
| Lipoprotein metabolism | Decreases HDL cholesterol (? androgen effects of 19-nortestosterone derivatives) | Increases HDL, VLDL, cholesterol (× 2)<br>Menopausal:– decreased LDL cholesterol and triglycerides | HDL:total cholesterol fall favours arterial diseases (relative risk 3–5×)<br>– haemorrhagic/thrombotic cerebral events<br>– ischaemic heart disease<br>– hypertension |
| Hypercoaguability | | Functional anti-thrombin III deficiency — associated with blood groups A, B, AB.<br>Increased clotting factors and platelet coaguability.<br>Decreased fibrinolytic activity | Venous thrombo-embolism relative risk: 3–10×<br><br>? arterial diseases |
| Protein synthesis | | Increased hormone binding globulins of cortisol, sex hormones, thyroid<br>Increased caeruloplasmin, transferrin, haptoglobulins, renin substrate globulins<br>Plasma amino acids and albumin decrease, but synthesis increased<br>Hepatic enzyme dysfunction | Increased concentration of bound hormones<br>Altered biochemical tests<br><br><br>Hypertension ? due to increased renin<br>Depression due to abnormal tryptophan metabolism<br>Biliary changes: cholelithias |
| Endocrine | | Stimulate calcitonin synthesis<br>May stimulate growth of prolactin secreting pituitary tumour<br>Hypothalamic-pituitary dysfunction | Prevent bone loss especially post menopausal<br>Pituitary infarction<br>Post-pill amenorrhoea, but rare as other causes of amenorrhoea are often found. |
| Carcinogenesis | prevent endometrial carcinoma | Endometrial changes<br>Breast duct changes<br>Liver cell changes | Endometrial carcinoma<br>Breast carcinoma<br>Liver tumours<br>Relative risk 3× |

5. Therapy should be stopped if complications develop or at presumed time of menopause (e.g. 40–45 years). It may be necessary to offer alternative forms of contraception, though most women are infertile after 48 years of age

*Indications for hormone replacement therapy*
 (i)  Gonadal failure in females
(ii)  Post-menopausal syndromes
    – alleviate symptoms — vasomotor phenomena, dyspareunia
    – preserve skeletal mass (i.e. retard osteoporosis)
    (*N.B.* oestrogens alone must not be used in post-menopausal women)

## ABNORMALITIES OF TESTICULAR FUNCTION

**Physiology** (Fig. 8.5)

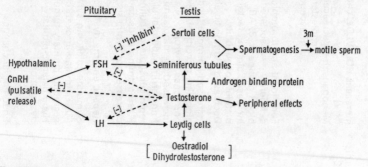

Fig. 8.5

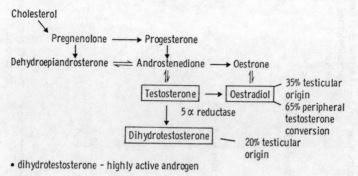

• dihydrotestosterone – highly active androgen

Fig. 8.6

*Leydig cells*
Synthesize sex steroids under influence of LH (Fig. 8.6).
- dihydrotestosterone — highly potent androgen mostly derived
  from peripheral conversion of testosterone

*Sertoli cells*
- essential for spermatogenesis
- source of nutrient for germinating cells in seminiferous tubules
- secrete:
    - androgen binding protein concentrates testosterone at
      tubules — ? stimulated by FSH
    - 'inhibin' polypeptide which selectively inhibits FSH secretion
    - Mullerian inhibitory factor causes ipsilateral Mullerian duct
      regression during fetal development
- essential for spermatogenesis

**Failure of testicular function (hypogonadism)**

*Causes*
Hypogonadotrophic hypogonadism (secondary failure with low
FSH/LH)
- hypothalamic dysfunction
    - GnRH deficiency e.g. Kallmans syndrome
    - tumours
    - irradiation
    - chronic illness/starvation
    - granulomatous disease
    - Prader-Willi syndrome
    - Laurence-Moon-Biedl syndrome
- pituitary failure
    - tumours
    - infarction
    - hypophysectomy
    - irradiation
    - granulomatous disease
    - hypothyroidism
Hypergonadotrophic hypogonadism (primary failure with elevated
FSH/LH)
- testicular disease
    - tumours
    - infarction; torsion, trauma etc.
    - surgery
    - agenesis
    - germ cell damage: radiation, cytoxics, mumps orchitis
    - tubular failure: Klinefelters, dystrophica myotonica
    - Leydig cell failure: alcohol, renal failure, malnutrition
    - cryptorchidism
    - autoimmune (anti-sperm antibodies)
    - idiopathic failure (old age)

- androgen deficiency
  - enzyme defects
  - testicular feminizing syndrome (androgen resistance)

*Clinical features*
- androgen deficiency during fetal development results in pseudohermaphroditism
- pubertal failure results in immature genitalia, lack of sexual and body hair, effeminate voice, skeletal span exceeds height by 5 cm, infertility, low libido + gynaecomastia
- androgen failure in developed adults results in impotence, low libido, and gradual loss of secondary hair
- features of associated disease

*Investigations*
- serum testosterone; semen analysis, karyotype if necessary
- serum LH — elevated in Leydig cell failure
- serum FSH — elevated in tubular-Sertoli cell failure
- low LH/FSH (see below)
- testicular biopsy in doubtful cases

*Treatment*
- primary failure is usually irreversible requiring replacement with testosterone. Parenteral depot preparations are preferred e.g. primotestone 250 mg i.m. monthly as oral absorption of testosterone is poor. Frequency of injection should aim to keep blood testosterone levels in normal range before next injection is due

*Idiopathic hypogonadotrophic hypogonadism*
- a disorder of the hypothalamus resulting in a variable deficiency of GnRH secretion (Fig. 8.7)
- can be inherited — autosomal dominant with variable genetic expression or genetically heterogenous

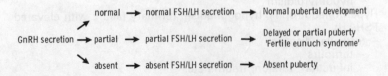

FSH/LH response to exogenous GnRH administration is variable and can improve with successive doses

**Fig. 8.7**

- associated with mid-line oro-facial abnormalities, olfactory dysfunction (Kallmans syndrome); olfactory neural links with hypothalamic gonadotrophin stimulatory neurons have been described

*Investigations*
- exclude pituitary/hypothalamic tumours with skull X-rays, and contrast enhanced CT scans, visual perimetry
- GnRH test and a combined pituitary function test as other anterior pituitary hormone deficiencies may be present e.g. growth hormone

*Treatment*
- human chorionic gonadotrophins (HCG) has 'LH-like' effect on Leydig cells to increase local testosterone secretion and concentration to promote spermatogenesis. Usual dose 2000–5000 i.u. twice weekly i.m. Pergonal 'FSH' can be added to HCG therapy
- pulsatile parenteral GnRH administered via portable infusion pumps has restored fertility in about 50%
- if fertility is not desired or impossible, give androgen replacement

*Follow-up*
- six month checks on serum testosterone, and semen analyses and dose of HCG adjusted; testicular pains or aggressive behaviour suggest HCG overdose
- prognosis for fertility is best in those with evidence of mild forms of the disorder e.g. isolated LH deficiency, presence of spermatozoa
- in some cases, gonadal function will be maintained after stopping HCG

**Undescended testicles**

*Normal descent*
- placental and fetal gonadotrophins influence descent
- descent guided by gubernaculum and is completed by 8 months of fetal life
- scrotal testes mature by age of 5 years

*Incidence*
- 3% have bilateral cryptorchidism at birth; unilateral cryptorchidism occurs in 12%
- 0.5% have bilateral cryptorchidism at age of 1 year with little chance of any subsequent descent

## Causes of 'missing' testicles
- retractile testicles — commonest cause
- cryptorchidism
  - intra-abdominal
  - maldescent
  - ectopic
- intersex states (see p. 144)
- atrophic testis in scrotum — often unilateral

## Risks of undescended testicles
- torsion/trauma
- irreversible dysfunction especially spermatogenesis
- malignant change after puberty especially if intra-abdominal

## Management
- children best examined in warm bath as retractile testis are more easily demonstrated
- careful genital examination to exclude intersex states
- atrophic scrotal testis, or ectopic should be carefully palpated

## Treatment
- HCG 2000 i.u. i.m. twice weekly may aid descent in some. Precocious puberty may be precipitated by HCG
- orchidopexy should not be delayed beyond the age of 5 years especially if bilateral cryptorchidism is present
- intra-abdominal testicular tissue can be demonstrated by giving 2000–5000 i.u. of HCG i.m. and observing rises of serum testosterone and oestradiol over the next 3 days. Intra-abdominal testicular tissue should be removed as malignant change can occur
- sialastic 'testicles' may be substituted in scrotal sac if orchidectomy necessary

## Prognosis for fertility
- excellent for unilateral cryptorchidism but if delay in bringing down testicle then spermatogenesis failure may occur in other (descended) testicle
- delay in orchidopexy for bilateral cryptorchids after the age of 5 results in infertility in 50%
- adults with bilateral cryptorchidism are usually infertile

## Follow-up
- essential for those being observed for spontaneous descent, repeated genital examination performed each visit
- those who have had bilateral orchidectomy will need androgen therapy at pubertal age, and change of 'sialastic testicle' size

**Gynaecomastia**

*Definition*
- unilateral or bilateral proliferation of glandular breast tissue in male
- multiple factors control normal breast development:

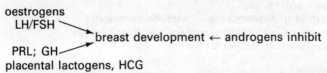

oestrogens
LH/FSH
            breast development ← androgens inhibit
PRL; GH
placental lactogens, HCG

*Causes*
There is some overlap of mechanisms.
- disturbed pituitary hormone secretion (gynaecomastia is often transient)
  - pubertal (can persist)
  - re-feeding
  - renal dialysis
  - tuberculosis treatment
  - hypo/hyperthyroidism
  - acromegaly
  - diabetes mellitus
- increased oestrogen + decreased androgen effect
  - adrenal carcinoma
  - primary testicular failure
    - tumours
    - cryptorchidism
    - agenesis e.g. Klinefelter's
    - radiation, surgery, cytotoxics
    - orchitis
  - testicular feminizing syndrome
  - hypogonadotrophic hypogonadism
  - liver disease
  - decreased sex hormone binding globulins
- increased placental lactogens, HCG etc.
  - some oat cell carcinoma
  - pinealoma
  - chorionepithelioma etc.
- drugs:
  - androgen antagonists:
    - spironolactone
    - cyproterone
    - cimetidine
  - 'Oestrogen' effect
    - digitalis
    - oestrogens
    - griseofulvin

- hypothalamo-pituitary effects
  - phenothiazines
  - antidepressants
  - metochlopramide
  - methyldopa

*Clinical features*
- if painful gynaecomastia — exclude carcinoma
- features of associated disorders e.g. liver disease, hypogonadism, testicular tumours etc.

*Investigations*
- HCG/oestrogens
- liver function tests
- thyroid hormone levels
- exclude hypogonadism
- karyotype if necessary
- chest X-ray; skull X-ray

*Treatment*
- treatment of cause may bring some reversal of gynaecomastia
- mastectomy is indicated for cosmetic or diagnostic reasons

## DISORDERS OF SEXUAL DIFFERENTIATION

### Normal sex differentiation (Fig. 8.8)
- gonadal agenesis results in female phenotype (infertile) irrespective of genotype
- gene locus on short arm of Y chromosome may control expression of the H–Y antigen via a further locus on the Y or another chromosome (H–Y antigen can occur in absence of Y chromosome)
- H–Y antigen acts on specific receptors on the bipotential (indifferent) gonad which then differentiates into testicle
- androgen deficiency or resistance will result in female external genitalia
- exposure of female embryo to androgen at critical stage of development results in male external genitalia

### Abnormal sex differentiation (Table 8.3)

### Principles of management
- undescended gonads of intersex states are especially prone to malignant change (50% incidence if containing 'Y' chromosome), and should be actively sought and excised
- behavioural and physical sexual development overrides genotypic sex when assigning sexual identity with hormone or plastic surgery

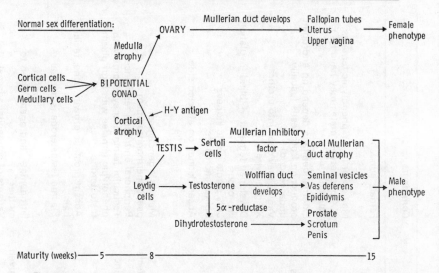

**Fig. 8.8**

**Sex chromosomal abnormalities** (Table 8.4)
- absent X chromosome incompatible with life; e.g. 45Y- lethal
- two X-chromosomes required for ovarian survival; single X results in germ cell death and streak gonad
- in mosaicism e.g. 47XXY/46XY, cells with Y chromosome differentiate into testicular tissue and other into ovaries ie. true hermaphroditism can occur

## DISORDERS OF PUBERTY

Normal puberty: mechanism of onset not known (Fig. 8.9).
Physical changes in puberty (due to sex steroids) (Table 8.5).

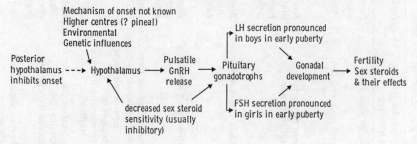

**Fig. 8.9**

**Table 8.3** Abnormal sex differentiation

| Developmental abnormality | Internal genitalia | External genitalia | Comments |
|---|---|---|---|
| Gonadal agenesis | Female (fallopians, uterus) no ovary | Female | Female eunuchs |
| Absent H–Y antigen | Female | Female | May occur in XY phenotypic females (XX phenotypic males may have H–Y antigen) |
| Absent Mullerian inhibitory factor | Female on deficient side, male on normal side. Female on both sides if defect bilateral | Variable male-hypospadias female | External genitalia depend on androgen production from testis (usually undescended) Vagina may open into urethra XY genotype |
| Mullerian duct agenesis | Absent or rudimentary uterus fallopians normal ovary | Hypoplastic | Developed females — 'blind' ovulation can occur 30% single pelvic kidneys Spinal anomalies |
| Wolffian duct agenesis | Absent epididymis, vas, seminal vesicles on affected side | Male | Absent kidney on affected side |
| Testosterone deficiency (17-dehydrogenase defect) Testosterone resistance – endogenous – cyproterone therapy to mother | Intraabdominal testis No vas, etc. | Variable – labioscrotal defects – hypospadias – female with 'blind' vagina | Male (XY genotypes) pseudohermaphroditism Peripheral androgen resistance Testicular feminizing syndrome with phenotypic females with high plasma testosterone |
| Dihydrotestosterone deficiency (5 δ-reductase deficiency) | Male Testis — spermatogenesis present | Small phallus Urogenital sinus | Absent prostatic growth, acne, facial hair Plasma testosterone is normal |
| Androgen exposure of female embryo | Female | Male tendency Clitoromegaly if given late | Iatrogenic — androgens given to mother Variants of congenital adrenal hyperplasia |

**Table 8.4** Sex chromosomal abnormalities

| Karyotype | % Birth incidence | Gonads | Habitus | Associated abnormalities |
|---|---|---|---|---|
| 45XO (Turners) | 0.04 of females | Fibrous streaks (fertility occurs in 45XO/46XX mosaics) | Female — retarded secondary sexual development Shield like chest Webbed neck Short metacarpals | Cardiovascular e.g. coarctation, septal defects, hypertension, colour blindness, ptosis, lymphatic aplasia, telangiectasia, renal abnormalities |
| 47XXX | 0.07 of females | Fertile ovary | Developed female | Mental retardation |
| 48XXXX etc | Rare | Streak gonad | Undeveloped female | Mental retardation |
| 47XXY (Klinefelter's) | 0.14–0.2 of males | Seminiferous tubular atrophy, variable Leydig cell function; no spermatogenesis Testis-hard, <2 cm diam. Cryptorchid | Eunuchoid male 50% gynaecomastia | Mental retardation Psychopathy Diabetes mellitus |
| 47XYY | 0.2 of males | Normal testis, fertile | Tall, severe acne Radio-ulnar synostosis | ? Criminal behaviour Mental retardation |
| Mosaics/ chimera e.g. 46XY/46XX | Rare | Coexistent testicular and ovarian tissues | Male to female often indeterminate | Mixed blood group etc. |

**Table 8.5**

|  | Boys | Girls |
| --- | --- | --- |
| Mean age of onset | 11.5 | 12.9 |
| Earliest changes | Testicular enlargement, scrotal rugosity, pubic hair, penile growth, pigmentary changes, accelerated skeletal growth | Breast buds, vulval growth, pubic hair, pelvic bone growth, linear growth |
| Later changes | Prostatic, seminal vesical development; male scalp, body hair distribution, laryngeal enlargement — voice change, male psyche, potency, epiphysial fusion | Menstruation, breast growth, pigmented nipples, vaginal, uterine growth and secretions, female body hair configuration, epiphysial fusion |

**Precocious puberty**

*Definition*
Puberty < age 10 boys; < age 8 girls
- true precocious puberty: gonadotrophins induce normal gonadal maturation
- pseudo-precocious puberty: extra-gonadal sex steroids suppress gonads

*Incidence*
- rare — male: female 1:3. 10% are familial
- 90% girls have idiopathic true precocity i.e. no cause found
- 25% boys have idiopathic true precocity — pseudoprecocity commonest cause

*Causes*
- hypothalamic dysfunction (?loss of inhibitory influences)
  - idiopathic
  - tumours, pinealoma
  - hamartoma (can secrete GnRH)
  - post infective — meningitis, encephalitis, toxoplasmosis
  - hypothyroidism
  - others e.g. polyostotic fibrous dysplasia, tuberose sclerosis
- congenital adrenal hyperplasia (CAH) (commonest cause in males — present at birth)

- testosterone/oestrogen source
  - iatrogenic
  - adrenal tumour (usually malignant)
  - testicular (Leydig cell) and ovarian (Thecal cell etc.) tumours
- HCG exposure (LH-like effect)
  - tumour secretion: chorionepithelioma, hepatoma, hepatoblastoma
  - iatrogenic e.g. for cryptorchidism

*Clinical features*
- early pubertal changes occur with gonadal enlargement in true precocity
- virilization in girls suggests adrenal carcinoma
- early epiphysial fusion results ultimately in short stature i.e. bone age advanced
- visual field defects, diabetes insipidus, seizures, bulimia etc. suggest intra-cranial cause

*Investigations*
- serum sex steroids elevated in all cases
- serum LH, FSH are elevated with intact GnRH responses in true precocity, but are suppressed in pseudoprecocity
- urinary 17-oxosteroids are elevated but suppressed by dexamethasone in C.A.H.; failure to suppress 17-oxosteroids suggest adrenal carcinoma
- urinary HCG
- laparoscopy useful in detecting ovarian pathology
- radiology:  skull X-ray; CT head scanning but may miss small hamartomas
            adrenal visualization: CT scan,
            angiography etc. if tumour suspected

*Treatment*
- pseudoprecocious puberty may be ameliorated with surgery, radiotherapy or drugs
- most intra-cranial causes are surgically inaccessible and medical therapy favoured
- gonadotrophin secretion can be suppressed with progestogens
  — medroxyprogesterone, danazol etc. but skeletal maturation unaffected
- GnRH agonists which down-regulate pituitary gonadotrophin secretion combined with cyproterone acetate (peripheral androgen antagonist) have been used

*Follow-up*
- important in boys where cause likely to emerge during follow-up

## Delayed puberty

*Definition*
- absence of early pubertal changes by age 15 years in boys and 14 years in girls

*Causes*
Commonest cause:
- constitutional (+ family history of delayed puberty)
Common causes: (? functional disturbance of hypothalamic pituitary axis)
- systemic/chronic diseases
  - renal
  - cardiac
  - respiratory
  - hepatic
  - etc.
- malabsorption, starvation
- psycho-social stress
Rare causes:
- hypothalamic-pituitary diseases
- gonadal diseases
- congenital adrenal hyperplasia
- hypothyroidism
- diabetes
- chromosomal/developmental abnormalities

*Clinical features*
- associated disorder may be obvious
- eunuchoidal skeletal proportions suggest gonadal failure
- markedly short stature suggests associated GH deficiency, hypothyroidism, Turner's syndrome etc.
- genitalia examination — chromosomal/intersex states should be considered
- olfactory function should be assessed (Kallmans syndrome)
- visual field defects should be excluded

*Investigations*
- exclude associated diseases
- serum sex steroids, serum T4 and T3
- serum gonadotrophins
- combined pituitary function tests
- skull radiology and CT scanning
- bone age (wrists etc.) usually retarded
- karyotype — to exclude Turner's, Klinefelter's, mosaics etc.

*Treatment*
- family history of delayed puberty, bone age > 14 years or < 2 years behind chronological age, and absence of obvious causes suggests constitutional delay; reassurance and observation will suffice in most
- if no sign of puberty by age 16 years, more detailed investigations may be required to exclude above causes
- HCG i.m. 1500–3000 i.u. twice weekly for about 6–12 months will induce pubertal changes if gonads are intact, and fertility maintained
- neurosurgical treatment may be deferred until spontaneous puberty has occurred as induction of puberty more difficult after neurosurgery
- primary gonadal failure, where fertility impossible will require monthly parenteral testosterone in male or oestrogens + progesterone in females using incremental dose regimens to mimic normal puberty in both
- growth hormone deficiency must be excluded as genetic growth potential may be limited by early epiphysial closure induced by sex steroids

## ABNORMALITIES OF STEROID SYNTHESIS

### Normal steroid metabolism (Fig. 8.10)

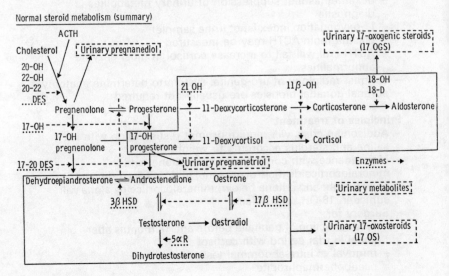

Fig. 8.10

- most enzyme deficiencies are inherited as autosomal recessive. Compensatory ACTH induces adrenal hypertrophy 4–10× normal. Excess sex steroid production will suppress pituitary gonadotrophin secretion
- accumulation and diversion of metabolites will occur proximal to enzyme defect, while deficiency will occur distally. Adrenal, gonadal and peripheral steroid synthesis can be involved
- clinical presentation determined by
  - site of enzyme defect
  - degree of enzyme deficiency i.e. complete or partial
- may present as:
  - adreno-cortical insufficiency — usually 1 week after birth birth
  - intersex state/virilization/male pseudohermaphrodite
  - puberty — precocity/failure
  - hypertension

CAH should be considered with any of above features, especially when present at birth and actively excluded.
(see Table 8.6 for specific associated syndromes)

**Investigations**
- karyotype required to establish sex when ambiguous genitalia present
- serum and urinary steroid profiles (see Table 8.6); can be predicted (see Fig. 8.10)
  - dexamethasone: suppression of urinary metabolites is diagnostic
  - 11-oxygenation index (spot urine sample)
  - plasma renin/ACTH may be measured
  - ACTH i.m. will fail to increase cortisol in most enzyme abnormalities
- contrast radiology of uro-genital system to determine anatomy
- adrenal/gonadal biopsies are usually not required

**Principles of treatment**
- Addisonian crisis will require prompt resuscitation with i.v. saline and steroids according to weight of baby
- Maintenance with cortisol (or prednisolone) and mineralocorticoids (fludrocortisone) in doses according to body weight and criteria below; mineralocorticoids alone will suffice in 18-OH, 18D defects
- Surgery for:
  - reconstruction of genitalia before age 18 months after suitable trial period with cortisol
  - removal of intra-abdominal testis in male pseudohermaphrodite

| Enzyme deficiency | Clinical features | Aids to diagnosis |
| --- | --- | --- |
| 20-hydroxylase (20–OH)<br>22-hydroxylase (22–OH)<br>20–22 desmolase (20–22 Des) | Adrenal insufficiency (most die soon after birth)<br>Female external genitalia<br>Pigmentation | ACTH +++<br>Cortisol low |
| 3-β-hydroxy dehydrogenase (3βHSD) | Adrenal insufficiency<br>Males — ambiguous genitalia<br>Females — virilization (peripheral conversion of dehydroepiandro-sterone to testosterone) | ACTH +<br>Cortisol low<br>Pregnanediol ++<br>17–OS ++ |
| 17–OH<br>17–20 Des<br>17–β HSD | Hypertension + hypokalaemia<br>Males — pseudohermaphroditism<br>Females — pubertal failure | ACTH + FSH/LH +<br>11-deoxycorticosterone ++<br>Plasma renin low, aldosterone + <br>urinary pregnandiol and aldosterone ++ |
| 21–OH<br>Commonest at birth 1/50000–1/5000<br>1/50 = gene carrier | Severe — adrenal insufficiency (salt losing) at 5–8 days 30% — females may appear to have male external genitalia or virilization<br>males — precocious puberty | ACTH ++<br>Plasma renin ++<br>Pregnanetriol ++<br>17–OS ++ |
| 11–β OH | Moderate hypertension<br>Males — precocious puberty<br>Females — virilization | ACTH ++<br>11-deoxycorticosterone ++<br>11-deoxycortisol ++<br>17-OS ++ (dexamethasone suppresses) |
| 18–OH<br>18-D-dehydrogenase | Hypotension — salt loss marked | Corticosterone ++<br>Aldosterone low<br>Plasma renin elevated |
| 5α-reductase (5αR) | Males — small phallus, urogenital sinus<br>– absent secondary sexual hair<br>– no prostatic growth<br>– spermatogenesis intact | Testosterone normal |

+ = elevated

## Follow up

Essential and may be life long:
- blood pressure, growth, bone age, with ACTH, serum and urinary steroids maintained within normal range on minimal dose of corticosteroids
- androgen and oestrogen therapy may be required at puberty with some enzyme defects
- it may be possible to stop steroids in developed males with mild enzyme deficiency but females should continue as virilization may occur
- corticosteroids will need to be increased during 'stress' circumstances; patients should carry s.o.s. alert devices

## Prognosis

- 20-OH, 27-OH, 20–22 Des, 3β-HSD associated with low survival rates despite early initiation of therapy
- fertility more likely if treatment early, but 17-OH deficiency confers infertility despite appropriate steroid replacement

## Gonadal endocrine tumours

| Testicular tumours | Ovarian tumours |
|---|---|
| Germ cell (HCG) seminoma embryonal — teratoma mixed seminoma/embryonal choriocarcinoma gonadoblastoma (occurs intersex states) | Germ cell (HCG) embryonal teratoma etc. choriocarcinoma gonadal blastoma (can also secrete human placental lactogen; steroids, calcitonin, thyroid hormones, etc.) |
| Interstitial/Leydig (androgens) | Interstitial/hilar/Leydig (androgen) Arrhenoblastoma, Sertoli-Leydig, theca granulosa (oestrogen, rarely progesterone) luteal (progesterone) |
| Adrenal rests (cortisol, androgens) | Adrenal rests (cortisol, androgen) |
| Stromal tumours e.g. fibroma | Stromal tumours |
| Secondaries | Secondaries |

(          ) = secreted hormone

- many 'silent' tumours may secrete inactive gonadotrophin subunits
- in some cases, tumour-secreted steroid precursors are converted to more active hormones peripherally
- germ cell tumours are:
  - highly malignant
  - younger age range, often prepubertal
  - associated with ectopic testicular tissue
- most commonly present as testicular or abdominal mass

*Clinical endocrine syndromes*
- virilization/hirsutes
- gynaecomastia
- precocious puberty
- hypogonadism/primary and secondary amenorrhoea
- thyrotoxicosis/carcinoid — extremely rare

*Investigations*
- see above syndromes in appropriate sections
- serum HCG (more sensitive than pregnancy test), testosterone, oestrogens FSH, LH
- urinary 17-OS may be elevated but not suppressible with dexamethasone
- laparoscopy — but small 'active' tumours may be missed
- venous sampling — best guide to source and activity of intra-abdominal tumours
- testicular biopsy; endometrial biopsy — hyperoestrogenism predisposes to carcinoma

*Treatment*
- germ cell tumours are excised and course of chemotherapy given as most are resistant to radiotherapy — prognosis variable
- seminomas are exceptionally sensitive to radiotherapy and have best prognosis (5 year survival 95%)

# 9. Pineal gland

- Develops from ependymal cells of 3rd ventricle
- Pineal cells (pinealocytes) are secretory — served by fenestrated endothelium (blood brain barrier is absent)
- In lower vetebrates, pineal is light sensitive with connections to brain
- In man pineal innervated by post-ganglionic sympathetic fibres from superior cervical sympathetic chain — linked to optic tract via retinohypothalamic tract and may relay non-conscious perception of light and dark

## PHYSIOLOGY

- In animals pineal sensitive to earth strength magnetic fields ? navigation function
- In man pineal is major source of melatonin; biogenic amines, releasing hormones e.g. GnRH, and other hormones (e.g. HCG) are also present
- Role of pineal in man is speculative
  *Melatonin* (Fig. 9.1)

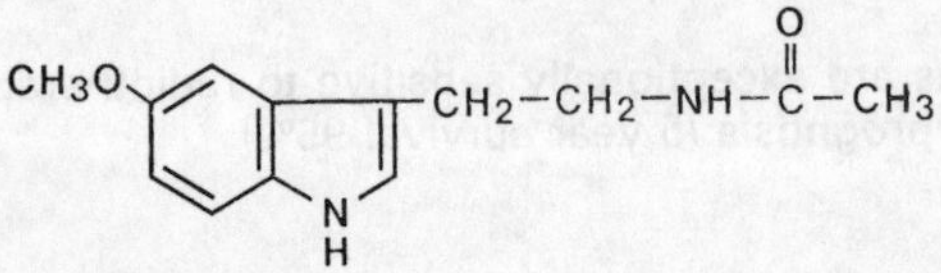

$$CH_3O\text{—} \quad \text{—}CH_2\text{—}CH_2\text{—}NH\text{—}\overset{\displaystyle O}{\overset{\displaystyle \|}{C}}\text{—}CH_3$$

**Fig. 9.1**

- synthesized from tryptophan
- N-acetyltransferase controls rate of melatonin synthesis
- secretion highest at night, suppressed by environmental light
- specific inhibitor of gonadotrophin secretion — even after GnRH
- ? regulates circadian rhythms

- ? role in control of onset of puberty — increased pre-puberty
- melatonin also increased by exercise, stress
- nocturnal melatonin secretion diminishes with age
- melatonin injections in man cause drowsiness

**Pineal calcification**
- Calcific nodules (acervuli) form in matrix secreted by pinealocytes
- Starts early and is common by 2nd decade
- Does not interfere with pineal function

**Pineal tumours**
- Germinomas
    - commonest tumours involving pineal
    - arise from germ cell rests in pineal
    - metastasize to spinal cord
    - are radiosensitive
- Pineal parenchymal tumours
    - Pinealocyte tumours of varying differentiation (true pinealomas)
    - Glial tumours
- Male preponderance

**Clinical effects of pineal tumours**
- Expansion effects
    - 3rd ventricle and floor of hypothalamus — hypogonadism, DI and optic atrophy
    - internal hydrocephalus
    - ocular effects (upward gaze palsy, light areflexia, papilloedema etc.)
- Endocrine effects
    - Precocious puberty due to pineal tumours is mainly seen in males
    - Precocious puberty is caused by:
        - destruction of 'inhibitory' structures in hypothalamus
        - secretion of HCG by pineal tumours e.g. teratoma

# 10. Ectopic hormone secretion

## Definition
Hormone secretion from neoplastic cells arising from non-endocrine tissue

## Mechanisms
- ? arise from diffuse endocrine system of cells of neural crest origin with:
  - cytochemical characteristics — amine precursor uptake decarboxylation (APUD)
  - common enzyme — neuron-specific enolase
- ? de-differentiation of cells during neoplasia

## Causes (Table 10.1)

**Table 10.1** Ectopic hormone secretion from tumours

| Hormone | Tumour | Clinical effects |
|---|---|---|
| *Releasing hormones or factors* | | |
| Corticotrophin releasing factor | Lung carcinoma Carcinoid | Hypokalaemic alkalosis, Cushing's syndrome |
| Growth hormone releasing factor | Lung carcinoma Carcinoid | Acromegaly |
| *Anterior pituitary* | | |
| 31K Precursor products e.g. ACTH, β-LPH, MSH CLIP, Endorphins | Lung carcinoma Thymoma Islet carcinoma Carcinoid Medullary thyroid carcinoma Phaeochromocytoma | Hypokalaemic alkalosis Cushing's syndrome in lowgrade malignancies Pigmentation |
| GH | ? Lung & gastric carcinoma | Arthropathy |
| PRL | Lung, gastric, breast & renal | Gynaecomastia |

| | | |
|---|---|---|
| Gonadotrophins (HCG, α & β subunits) | Lung, gastric, breast, islet and hepatic carcinomas Carcinoid | Gynaecomoasia Precocious puberty |
| *Posterior pituitary* Vasopressin, Oxytocin and Neurophysin | Lung carcinoma Carcinoid tumours | Dilutional hyponatraemia |
| *Others* Erythropoietin | Renal carcinoma Hepatic carcinoma Cerebellar haemangioma Uterine tumours GI tumours | Polycythaemia |
| PTH and PTH-like hormones | Renal carcinoma Squamous cell lung carcinoma | Hypercalcaemia |
| Calcitonin | Lung & breast carcinoma carcinoid, pancreatic tumours, phaeochromocytoma myeloid leukaemia | Absent |
| Somatostatin | Lung carcinoma Medullary thyroid carcinoma | Usually absent |
| Gastrin | Lung carcinoma Ovarian tumour | Usually absent |
| Insulin and glucagon | Lung carcinoma Carcinoid | Usually absent |
| VIP | Lung carcinoma | Diarrhoea |
| Somatomedin | Mesenchymal & adrenal tumours | Hypoglycaemia |
| Bombesin | Lung carcinoma Medullary thyroid carcinoma | Absent/unknown |

**Clinical features**
- Will depend on the quantity and activity of hormone secretion
- Many tumours have been shown to secrete biologically inactive hormone precursors
- If tumour is highly malignant, clinical features may not have time to develop, though metabolic abnormalities may be severe, e.g. lung carcinomas secreting ACTH may cause profound hypokalaemic alkalosis, but Cushing's syndrome usually not seen

**Diagnosis**
- Exclude commoner causes of endocrine syndrome
- Hormone responses to usual stimulation or suppression may be absent
- Selective venous catheterization may demonstrate increased hormone secretion from suspected site of tumour
- Hormone precursors or other hormones e.g. calcitonin may be secreted from the same tumour
- Clinical or biochemical remission of endocrine abnormality with removal of tumour
- Return of endocrine abnormality if tumour recurs
- Cytochemical evidence of hormone production in tumour cells
- Hormone secretion in tumour cell culture

**Treatment**
- As for underlying tumour — removal may reverse endocrine abnormalities
- If tumour not located, treat endocrine disorder symptomatically and maintain follow up of patient as tumour may declare itself